THE COMPLETE
PREGNANCY
WORKBOOK

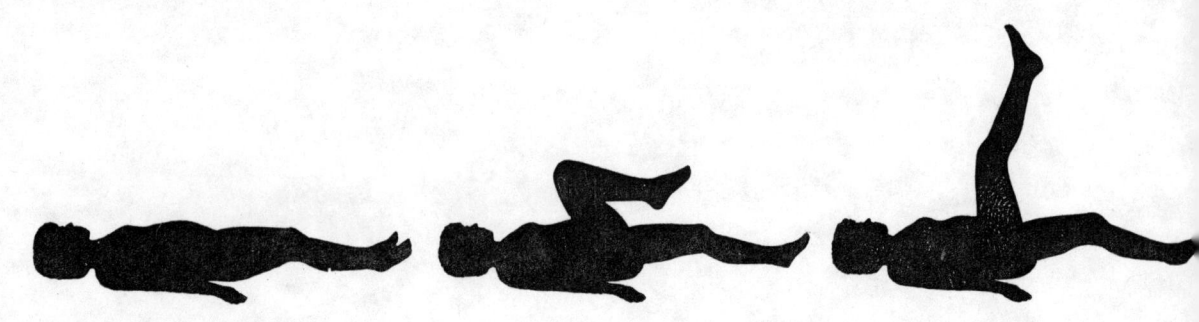

THE COMPLETE PREGNANCY WORKBOOK

A GUIDE FOR PARENTS-TO-BE

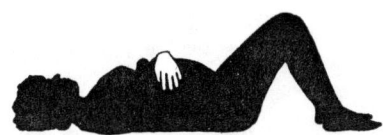

PHILIP D. SLOANE, M.D.
SALLI BENEDICT, M.P.H.
MELANIE MINTZER, M.D.

Illustrations by Thomas G. Waldrop

ALGONQUIN BOOKS OF CHAPEL HILL
1986

Algonquin Books of Chapel Hill
Post Office Box 2225
Chapel Hill, North Carolina 27515–2225

Printed in the United States of America.

Grateful acknowledgment is made to Grosset & Dunlap, Inc.,
for permission to reprint passages from *The Birth Diary* by
Sheila Kitzinger, published by The Stonesong Press, © 1980 by Sheila Kitzinger.

I S B N 0–912697–23–7

To our children,
Jesse and Jacob,
Jason and Gwendolyn,
and to Sidney and Florence Mintzer

Contents

Checklists and Worksheets

Preface

Being the father of my two boys has been the most reward-ing and challenging part of my life. As a family physician who provides obstetric care, I believe that well-informed patients are happier, less anxious, and therefore less likely to have problems during pregnancy. Nevertheless, I find that I finish an office visit without covering all the areas I would like to discuss with pregnant patients and their families. This book devel-oped from my desire to tell my patients everything they wanted to know about pregnancy, and to present options and choices to them in a straightforward way.

Salli Benedict, the mother of two children and a health educator, joined me in developing the book. We began by interviewing women during pregnancy and after childbirth to find out what they wanted to learn from books on pregnancy and from their physicians. We then organized topics according to when they are usually discussed during pregnancy. To make the learning process more active and personal, we chose a workbook format. Thus we hope to provide information in a way that will help you raise questions and, ulti-mately, participate more fully in your pregnancy, delivery, and par-enting experience.

We first wrote the workbook in 1982, and printed it for use by patients in our practice. As time went by, our readers told us it had helped them as we had hoped, so we began to think about revising it for a wider audience. Before doing so, we conducted a second series of interviews, this time talking to women who had used the workbook. We used their comments to revise and expand the original workbook. In these efforts we were joined by Melanie Mintzer, a family physician with a significant background and in-terest in women's health. You are holding the result of our efforts.

We sincerely hope that it provides you with information that will help make your pregnancy the best it can possibly be.

There are a few general comments I would like to make about the workbook:

- We have tried diligently to present facts, not opinions, whenever possible.
- We have tried to give you tools that will help you participate in the decisions involved in your care.
- We have tried to write the book not just for mothers-to-be, but for anyone who is interested in pregnancy and childbirth.
- Because doctors are not the only professionals who provide prenatal care or deliver babies, we use the term "health-care provider" to refer to the doctor, midwife, or any other individual who may provide care during pregnancy.
- We have chosen the term "partner" rather than "husband" or "wife" because some pregnancies take place outside of traditional marriages. We hope that our readers will not be confused by this wording. Where applicable, we have used non-sexist terminology such as "he or she."
- We have divided our readings into five parts, with three of the parts corresponding to early, middle, and late pregnancy, because pregnancy tends to have a different feel early on, in the middle, and near its end. The readings we have included in each part reflect what our patients have needed to know or have seemed most interested in at a given stage of pregnancy.

Finally, we would like to acknowledge with our thanks those individuals whose special help, guidance, and support enabled us to bring this book into a publishable form: Jean Cates, RN; Bob Gwyther, MD; Mike Fleming, MD; Trish Barron, MPH; Heidi Bruninghaus, RN; Watson Bowes, MD; Robert Cefalo, MD; Peter Curtis, MD; Jo Ann Crowe, RN; Diane Asbill, RN; Maggie Sloane; Kat Seiple; Jeff Bass; Jerome Shoaf; Kay Lovelace, MPH; Henry Fuchs; Jo Cohen; Marta Fuchs; Julianne Frey; Judy Crow; Julia Lyles; Marty Hawks; Margaret Morse; Susan Mabie; Jim Wainer; Louis Rubin; Joyce Kachergis; Garrett Epps; Paul Betz; and the Family Practice residents and the prenatal patients of the Family Practice Center at the University of North Carolina–Chapel Hill.

Philip D. Sloane, MD
January 1985

PART I

Before You Get Pregnant

1 Making the Decision

What's it like to have a child? Do I want to become a parent? Will I be a good parent? These questions are asked every day by thoughtful men and women. Posing such questions is a relatively new occurrence, for it was assumed in the past that everyone who was able would bear children. Only recently, with the development of effective birth control, has the decision not to have children been available to couples. Making a conscious choice allows you to consider the pros and cons about an event that will shape your life for decades to come.

Should You Have a Child?

How do you decide about having a child? Studies of couples clearly show that the decision is only partially a rational one. When discussing their reasons for having children, parents-to-be talk about such things as fulfillment, leaving something in the world that will live on after they die, expectations they were given while growing up, and personal attraction toward children. When you think about what it's like to be a parent, your strongest images will probably be memories of your own childhood. In fact, you are more likely to be happy as a parent if you have favorable memories of your childhood and of your parents' roles.

There are specific things about parenthood that you should think about when deciding to have a child. Being a parent takes time and involves responsibility. Once you start a family, your personal freedom is inevitably reduced. Parents see their lives as less spontaneous because deciding to do something requires making arrangements for an additional person, who often has routines, paraphernalia, and (when old enough to talk) opinions. And couples with children talk about having less time for their own relationship and about the slowing of their careers. But most parents don't dwell on the restrictions they have had to face; they speak favorably of the learning, sharing, and emotional aspects of parenthood. Many describe parenthood as the most valuable experience they've ever had, one they do not at all regret. So, regardless of the challenges it may pose, parenthood is immensely fulfilling.

If you and your partner disagree on whether or when to have children, you are not alone. It is common for couples to have different opinions and to struggle to reach a compromise. These differences should be resolved, however, before pregnancy is a fact and no longer a choice. A baby is best viewed as a shared experience, one entered into willingly by both partners. Single parenthood can be workable, but it is not ideal because of the demands it imposes on one individual. If you and your partner face and resolve the ambivalent feelings you each may have about parenthood, you will be more able to live comfortably with your decision—whatever it is.

In attempting to decide whether to become a parent, you should examine your relationship with your partner. Ask yourselves the following questions:

Do you disagree about . . .

the desire to have a child?
when to have a child?
whether one parent will stay home with the child full-time, and, if so, for how long?
what kind of religious upbringing to provide for a child?

As a couple, have you had major disagreements about . . .

finances?
sex relations?
proper behavior in public?
dealing with parents or in-laws?
household tasks?

Is your relationship . . .

unhappy?
fairly happy?
perfect?

Answer these questions as honestly as you can. In reviewing your responses, do you find significant unhappiness or dissatisfaction in any of part of your relationship? If so, you should reflect on the desirability of adding a new and stressful dimension—parenthood—to the situation. Sometimes a professional counselor can help solve the problems in the life you share with your partner before you decide to have a baby.

Single Parenting

Many women happily and successfully parent children alone, even though it can be difficult and frustrating. If you are a woman who has chosen to become a parent on your own, there are factors you should consider and concerns you will have that may not be addressed in this book. No matter how independent in spirit a person may be, hardly anyone can do without at least some emotional support. Parenting is hard work and—even when shared by two committed adults—a lot of responsibility. It will be particularly important for you to seek out support from friends, relatives, babysitters, and childcare facilities. You may want to look for or help establish a support group for single parents in your community.

Keep in mind, too, the need to consider who will be responsible for your child should something happen to you. You will want to consult with a lawyer about this. While some of your questions and concerns are unique to single mothers, and therefore beyond the scope of what we have to say, most of the information in this book will also apply to you.

Is There a Best Time in Life to Have Children?

Many people wonder whether there is a "best" time to begin or enlarge a family. Some medical researchers claim that the "ideal" age for maternity is between 20 and 30, because in that period of a woman's life the risk of medical complications is lowest. The timing of pregnancy is very much an individual matter, though. For example, a secure, prepared mother of 34 is more likely to have a healthy pregnancy and enjoy parenthood than a fearful, financially insecure woman of 24.

Most parents also wonder about how large a family is desirable and how closely one birth should follow another. Common sense tells us most of what we know about these topics: The more children there are and the closer together they come, the more expensive parenting becomes and the less time parents have to devote to each child. Waiting less than 12 months after childbirth to get pregnant leads to a higher chance of complications, including low birth weight and infant death. Teenage mothers, in particular, should space their children at least two years apart.

The best method of deciding whether to enlarge your family is to take a realistic look at your personal preferences and resources. Having more children around the house does result in more illness among family members, but not to an unmanageable degree. Intelligence scores are highest among children in small families, except in the case of single children, who do more poorly than those with one or two siblings.

The teenage years are an especially difficult time to have children. Teenage marriages have a high separation rate, and having children can add greatly to the stress the couple may already be experiencing. Among teenage mothers, the rates of anemia, high blood pressure, premature delivery, and caesarean section are higher. These medical factors make it particularly important for teenage parents to select a physician during the first three months of pregnancy and to keep their routine prenatal appointments.

At the other end of the age spectrum, 35 is now often said to be the limit beyond which pregnancy presents ever greater risks. But the dangers have been largely exaggerated, for health is more important than age in determining a woman's fitness to handle pregnancy. There are, however, several points to consider if you are thinking of having a baby when you are 35 or older:

● Women over 35 often make excellent parents. It is quite common for women in their thirties, who for career reasons had not wanted children, to feel ready to begin a family. These "late" mothers tend to have more self-confidence and maturity. Relatively undisturbed by the the everyday hassles of parenting, they seem to take special joy in their children.

● Prenatal care is particularly important for this age group. There is definitely a higher risk for mothers as age increases. The maternal death rate steadily rises from 9 per 100,000 at ages 25–29 to 66 per 100,000 after age 40. Older mothers are more prone to diabetes and hypertension. First mothers over 35 are more liable to experience labor difficulties, but that is not the case among older mothers who have had a previous child.

● Mothers-to-be aged 34 and older should have genetic counseling to discuss the likelihood of chromosomal birth defects, which increases with advancing maternal age. Down's Syndrome, a hereditary condition involving mental retardation and certain medical problems, is the most common of these birth defects. Table 1 shows the rates of birth defects in relation to the age of the mother.

**Table 1. How the Odds of Genetic Birth Defects
Increase with Age**

Mother's age	Approximate risk of all chromosomal abnormalities	Approximate risk of Down's Syndrome
30–34	1 in 650	1 in 900
35–39	1 in 100	1 in 300
40–44	1 in 50	1 in 100
> 44	1 in 20	1 in 50

For women who are at high risk for chromosomal defects, amniocentesis offers a relatively safe method of identifying babies with chromosomal abnormalities. (See page 35 for a discussion of amniocentesis.)

Unplanned Pregnancy

Carefully making a conscious, thoughtful decision to have a child is probably the best way to enter parenthood, but many pregnancies occur less intentionally. In fact, about one-third of births to married women and two-thirds of births to unmarried women were not intended at the time of conception. You are not alone if your pregnancy was an "accident." But you are likely to be happy with parenthood if, after considering the pros and cons of terminating the unplanned pregnancy, you make a conscious choice to accept and want the birth of a child. A surprise pregnancy can be disastrous, yet it can also become as welcome an occurrence as a carefully planned event.

Getting in Shape for Pregnancy

If you are considering having a child, you can make a successful pregnancy much more likely by getting yourself in the best physical shape possible. The time to do so is *before*, not after, you get pregnant.

If you are overweight, you are at higher risk for diabetes, hypertension, and certain complications. Pregnancy is not the time to diet; so, it is wise to lose unwanted pounds before trying to get pregnant, assuming that you can do so.

Also, it is preferable to start prenatal vitamins as soon as you decide to try to get pregnant. There is some evidence suggesting that folic acid supplements of 0.3 to 1.0 mg a day very early in pregnancy may help prevent certain defects of brain development.

Vigorous physical conditioning is not something to start during pregnancy, but continuing an exercise program is valuable. Women who are in excellent physical condition have fewer aches and pains during pregnancy and shorter labors. Being in shape improves your ability to "push" during labor, and that may preclude the need for a forceps delivery or, in some cases, a caesarean section.

The checklist on page 239 can serve as guide in determining what you should do before you choose to become pregnant.

RECOMMENDED RESOURCES

Boston Women's Health Book Collective. *Ourselves and Our Children*. New York: Random House, 1978. A book about parenting, which includes an excellent chapter on deciding to have children. Written in an anecdotal style, full of personal experiences and viewpoints.

Whelan, Elizabeth M. *A Baby? . . . Maybe*. New York: Bobbs-Merrill, 1976. The first book to explore in detail the considerations involved in deciding whether to have children.

2 Preparing for a Healthy Pregnancy

All prospective parents want their child to be healthy and normal at birth. However, a small percentage of babies (about 3 percent) are born with a significant birth defect. In this chapter, we will discuss birth defects and related complications of pregnancy as well as provide you with guidelines for protecting your baby from the causes of such painful problems.

When we talk about risks to the baby, it is important to emphasize that we do not have all the answers. In fact, only a small minority of birth abnormalities (between 18 and 40 percent, depending on the estimate) can be explained by known hazards. The advice given below offers you only a limited—though valuable—opportunity to safeguard the health of your unborn child.

Prepregnancy planning is particularly vital in the effort to protect against defects. The developing fetus is most sensitive to many known hazards during the first eight weeks of pregnancy. In other words, the critical period is before your first visit to the doctor and, often, before you are even sure you are pregnant. If there are changes that can be made in your life to reduce risks to an unborn child, the best time to make them is before getting pregnant.

Should You Have Genetic Counseling?

Some babies are born with birth defects or hereditary diseases that can be anticipated by genetic counseling and looked for in pregnancy by amniocentesis (see page 35). Most genetic diseases are rare, and for that reason only couples known to be at high risk are referred to a specialist for genetic counseling. The questions listed below will help you determine whether you should seek counseling of this kind.

For both parents-to-be:

Have you already had a child with a significant birth defect or a known hereditary disease, such as muscular dystrophy?

Do you suffer from a birth defect or hereditary disease?

Does any relative (parent or sibling) have a significant birth defect or known hereditary disease (including mental retardation)?

Is there any hereditary health problem that affects two or more family members, however distantly related?

Are you and your spouse first cousins or more closely related?

For the mother-to-be:

Are you 34 years of age or older?

Have you had two or more miscarriages and not yet had a child?

For the father-to-be:

Are you 55 years of age or older?

If you answered *yes* to any of the questions listed above, you may benefit from genetic counseling before attempting to have a child. Speak with your health-care provider about it.

The Rh Factor

The Rh factor is a term for certain components of the red blood cells of most people. Those who lack the Rh factor are called Rh-negative. If a pregnant woman is Rh-negative, and her unborn child is Rh-positive, antibodies from the mother may cross the placenta and destroy the baby's red blood cells, thus causing severe anemia. In order to make these antibodies, the mother has to have been exposed to Rh-positive blood cells, a process that usually happens during a delivery or miscarriage. In the past, many babies were born ill or died as a result of Rh problems, but this has become extremely rare. Today, virtually all Rh-negative women can anticipate a normal pregnancy and delivery as long as they see a physician regularly and keep to a routine of blood tests and treatment during prenatal care.

The medical advance that so dramatically improved the outlook for Rh-negative mothers is an injection called RhIg or RhoGAM. When given within 72 hours of a delivery or miscarriage, RhIg destroys any foreign blood cells that have gotten into the Rh-negative mother's bloodstream, thereby preventing the mother from making antibodies. If you are Rh-negative, the best preventive measure you can take is to make sure that you are given an injection of RhIg after each delivery or miscarriage (unless the baby is Rh-negative and therefore not capable of causing antibody formation).

It has now begun to be routine for many health-care providers to give Rh-negative mothers an additional RhIg injection at about the twenty-eighth week of pregnancy. This extra protective measure will probably soon become a regular practice in health-care services.

Genital Herpes

If you have genital herpes, you risk passing the disease on to your baby during childbirth. Transmission, though, can happen only if herpes sores are present at the time your baby is born. A woman with frequent herpes attacks is thus more likely to infect her baby than one who has very few attacks. Babies infected with herpes during childbirth can get very ill, and as many as half of them will die.

Herpes will not affect your ability to get pregnant. It also does not cause deformities in the baby unless your first attack occurs while you are pregnant. Even then, it very rarely creates difficulties. However, you cannot afford to be silent about the problem: if you have genital herpes, tell your health-care provider.

The current treatment for a pregnant woman with genital herpes is to have her undergo a pelvic examination every week during the last one or two months before the baby is due. During the examination, your health-care provider will look for herpes sores on your vulva, vagina, and cervix and will take either a Pap smear or a herpes culture, which can reveal herpes infections that cannot be seen.

When you go into labor, your health-care provider will review the last two weeks. If no sign of herpes has been observed—either by examination or in laboratory tests—and you have not been aware of any feelings that might warn of a herpes attack, it is safe for your baby to be born in the normal way. If signs of recent herpes are present, you should have a caesarean section.

As soon as your water breaks, your baby is no longer protected from herpes. At that time, or as soon as labor begins, a woman with herpes will need to contact her health-care provider. Often, a decision about performing a caesarean section will then have to be made.

If you have genital herpes, don't hesitate to discuss the situation with your health-care provider. The risk of problems is extremely low as long as you seek out and obtain the proper, timely preventive care.

Occupational Risks

The workplace is a common source of exposure to agents that can cause birth defects. Unfortunately, there is all too little known about the risks of exposure to occupational hazards during pregnancy. The following agents are known to cause deformities and other birth defects (see chapter 9 for details):

cadmium · lead · mercury · benzene

halogenated hydrocarbons: vinyl chloride, tetrachloroethylene, polychlorinated biphenyls (PCBs), etc.

anesthetic gases · carbon monoxide · x-rays · carbon disulfide

If any of the agents listed above are in the environment where you work, you should discuss the risks with your health-care provider before getting pregnant.

In particular, if you work around x-rays, you should request that your monitoring badge be read monthly to ensure that your exposure remains in the safe range. The recommended x-ray dosage limit for a pregnant woman is 1.5 rem.

Avoidable Environmental Risks

It may not be possible or practical for you to avoid certain potentially hazardous substances where you work, but there are risks to your body and your unborn child over which you can and should exercise control.

Smoking, for example, is a common environmental hazard you can avoid. Inhalation of tobacco smoke introduces into your body carbon monoxide, an unquestionably harmful agent. Babies born to smokers are typically smaller than those of non-smokers. But that is not nearly so much of a problem as the increased risk of death to the baby of a woman who smokes. Babies of light smokers are more likely to die during delivery; those of heavy smokers have a 35 percent higher mortality rate. Clearly, not smoking will be good for the health of your baby.

Alcohol is another environmental risk you can avoid. In fact, al-

cohol is probably the most important preventable cause of birth
defects. It can lead to a variety of problems, including reduced intelligence and mental retardation. While heavy drinkers (those
who have more than two drinks per day) and binge drinkers are
known to run a greater risk of bearing children with birth defects,
it is not known whether small amounts of alcohol cause subtle injury during certain critical developmental periods. For that reason,
some physicians recommend limiting the consumption of alcohol
to no more than two drinks in a day; others advise that pregnant
women avoid alcohol altogether during the first three months or
longer.

One more avoidable environmental risk should be mentioned
here. In the first trimester of pregnancy, hyperthermia—or high
body temperature—may cause serious birth defects, including
anencephaly (incomplete development of the brain). If you think
you are pregnant, avoid saunas and hot-tub immersions of longer
than 15 minutes and treat all fevers over 101° F with acetaminophen (Tylenol, Datril, etc.).

Rubella and Toxoplasmosis

Two of the infections known to cause serious birth defects are
largely preventable.

Rubella (German measles) is a mild virus infection than can
cause major problems in babies, including cataracts, glaucoma,
heart defects, deafness, and mental retardation. Though most
women have had a rubella shot or had the disease as children,
15 percent of women who become pregnant do not have immunity.
Some women are not immune because their rubella shots in childhood did not "take." Others were told they had German measles,
but had in fact some other virus. If you are not immune to rubella
and get the virus during the first three months of your pregnancy,
the chance of birth defects is between 10 and 50 percent, with the
risk being highest during the first month.

Rubella immunization is more effective now than it was years
ago, and it is quite safe. It should, however, be administered before
you get pregnant. The vaccine itself contains a live, though weak-
ened, strain of the virus and thus can infect the fetus if given during pregnancy. (This risk is minimal. Of 959 documented cases
in which the rubella vaccine was given to pregnant women, no
rubella-related birth abnormalities were found.) To protect yourself and your baby, you should have a blood test for rubella immu-

nity before you get pregnant. If you are not immune, get a rubella shot and wait three months before attempting to get pregnant.

Toxoplasmosis is another preventable infection. Caused by a small protozoan, it is a common illness among adults. In fact, by age 50, about half of all American women have had toxoplasmosis. Most people who contract the illness suffer from fever and chills and think they have the flu; it is so mild that it often goes unnoticed. If passed on to a fetus, however, toxoplasmosis can cause partial or complete blindness, mental retardation, and other serious birth defects.

Approximately six women in 1000 become infected with toxoplasmosis during pregnancy, and between one-sixth and one-third of them pass it on to the fetus. As the pregnancy progresses, the chance of an infected mother transmitting her illness to the fetus increases—from about 35 percent in the first trimester to 75 percent in the third trimester. On the other hand, damage to the fetus is more extensive the earlier in pregnancy the disease is contracted. Toxoplasmosis is therefore a potential concern during all nine months.

Many people develop toxoplasmosis by being around pet cats, which often carry the disease without becoming sick themselves. Cat litter is a particularly likely source of exposure, since infected cats excrete the organism in their stool. If you've had a cat for a while and it has toxoplasmosis, you are probably already immune to the disease—so don't worry about your pet. If you are anticipating pregnancy, or have already conceived, you should, however, avoid getting a new cat. At any stage in your pregnancy, you should have someone else in the household change the cat-litter box.

Raw meat can also be on occasion a source of toxoplasmosis. Make it a practice to eat only cooked meat.

Dangerous Drugs

One of the major controversies in prenatal care is the risk posed by drugs during pregnancy. (See chapter 9 for more details about the subject.) A few drugs are known to cause birth defects; some others are suspected sources of birth abnormalities; and many others are thought to be of no harm to the fetus. However, scientific tests have proven the safety of only a small number of drugs when used by pregnant women.

As a rule, avoid drugs during the time you are pregnant. If you are using a medication and cannot clearly determine its safety, speak with your health-care provider about it. If you are taking drugs on a regular basis for medical reasons and definitely need them, it is often best to continue them while you are pregnant.

Certain classes of drugs, however, are particularly risky to the fetus. These should not be used by a pregnant woman under any circumstances:

- **disulfiram (Antabuse)**—used in treating alcoholism

- **paramethadione and trimethadione**—two similar drugs used for some kinds of seizures

- **diethylstilbesterol**—a synthetic hormone

You should also know about the kinds of drugs that are strongly linked to birth defects or complications in pregnancy but which sometimes need to be given to a pregnant woman. Within some of the categories listed below (such as anticonvulsants), there are drugs that are relatively safe for you to take if you are carrying a child. However, you should *definitely* consult your physician if you are taking drugs in any of these categories and are considering getting pregnant:

- **drugs used in the treatment of cancer**
- **drugs used for epilepsy or seizures**
- **drugs such as coumadin that prevent blood clots** (blood thinners)
- **oral antibiotics for acne or related conditions**
- **tetracycline and related drugs**
- **reserpine** (a blood-pressure medication)
- **antidepressants**
- **tranquilizers, sedatives, or sleeping pills**
- **diuretics** ("water pills")

Anticipating and Minimizing Your Own Medical Risks

Keep in mind that a pregnancy involves the health of *two* individuals. If you are planning to become a mother, there are steps you can take to ensure your optimum health—as well as your baby's. As we mentioned earlier, you will want to get in shape for pregnancy by practicing good nutrition and by exercising regularly. Another important step is routine medical care. You should have a general physical and a Pap test within two years of getting pregnant. Beyond these measures, women in good overall health do not require special medical attention before becoming pregant. (Of course, once you know you are pregnant, you should go to a health-care provider for regular prenatal care.)

If you have significant medical problems, however, your health may be threatened by the stresses of pregnancy. Any woman with a chronic illness or disability needs to consult with her physician before she plans to bear a child. Also, any woman who has had previous obstetric problems will have to discuss with her physician whether it is now safe for her to carry a fetus and give birth. A prepregnancy visit can often predict medical problems and make it easier to remain healthy during pregnancy. If there are definite health risks to your getting pregnant, you should know about them *beforehand*. The accompanying box lists some of the medical problems requiring special consideration during pregnancy.

If Any of These Conditions Apply to You, Contact Your Physician BEFORE Getting Pregnant

Current medical problems	Previous obstetric problems
Diabetes	Surgery on the uterus
Thyroid disease	Severe bleeding after delivery
Congenital heart disease	Delivery of a premature infant
Chronic kidney disease	Preeclampsia
Hypertension	3 or more miscarriages
Cancer	Stillbirth
Paraplegia or hemiplegia	2 or more induced abortions
Any hereditary or chronic anemia or other blood disease	
A heart murmur due to previous rheumatic fever	

RECOMMENDED RESOURCE

Briggs, C. G., T. W. Bodendorfer, R. K. Freeman, and S. T. Yaffe. *Drugs in Pregnancy and Lactation.* Baltimore and London: Williams and Wilkins, 1983. The most comprehensive review to date of the available information on drugs and pregnancy. Designed as a reference work for health-care providers.

3 Getting Pregnant

Y ou and your partner have now decided that you'd like to become parents. You've done what you can to minimize potential health risks to yourself and the baby. You're ready to *get pregnant*. For most people, a whole new set of questions arises at this point—questions about fertility, contraception, and planning the sex of the child. In this chapter, we consider some of these common questions about the process of getting pregnant. We do not discuss how babies are made or sexual problems between couples, which are addressed in other kinds of publications. Instead, we assume that you and your partner are a heterosexual couple and are able to have normal sexual intercourse when you choose to. Starting at that point, here is some background to aid you as you attempt to get pregnant.

How Long Will It Take to Get Pregnant?

When a couple decides to have a child, it usually takes less than a year for the woman to conceive. In the case of 80 percent of couples who have had a previous child, the woman will conceive within nine months; and in 96 percent of such couples, conception will occur within three years. Of couples who have not had a previous child, the pregnancy rates are similar, but about 10 percent will not achieve their goal within three years.

Previous contraception has no effect on pregnancy rates, except for the birth-control pill, which delays conception for an average of one month. Of women who have no previous children and have used the pill, 75 percent will conceive within a year of trying to get pregnant. In comparison, 82 percent of women who have practiced other contraceptive methods will be pregnant within a year. By three years after attempting to get pregnant, 90 percent of women will conceive, regardless of what kind of contraception they once used. So, having taken the pill slightly delays but does not reduce your chance of getting pregnant.

If you have recently had a child, your fertility will be reduced, but even breastfeeding does not prevent pregnancy entirely. Women who do not breastfeed have their first ovulation at about the third month after childbirth. Among breastfeeding mothers, the first ovulation occurs at about the fifth month after childbirth, with fertility seeming to return when breastfeeding is reduced to fewer than four or five nursings a day. Thus, while there is a certain child-spacing effect from breastfeeding, modern contraceptive methods are more reliable.

If You Have Had a Previous Miscarriage

Couples who have gone through a miscarriage are naturally concerned about the possibility of their having a healthy baby. After a woman has had one miscarriage, she stands a normal chance of getting pregnant again, but the likelihood of her having another miscarriage is higher. Previous miscarriages without a successful pregnancy do reduce the possibility of ever carrying a pregnancy to term; but the odds remain in favor of success even after three consecutive miscarriages. The chance of eventually having a full-term baby is 76 percent if you have had one miscarriage, 74 percent after two miscarriages, and 68 percent after three miscarriages.

If You Become Pregnant While Using a Contraceptive

Some couples approach contraception casually, saying something like this: "We wouldn't really mind if we had a child, so we aren't as careful as we could be with our birth control." This approach is fine if you use the rhythm method or condoms, which are completely safe if used even when you are pregnant. Other methods, however, might pose a risk to the fetus. Thus, it would be preferable for you to decide to stop contraception and make a conscious effort to get pregnant rather than use contraceptives only on occasion.

Almost all contraceptives seem remarkably safe if accidentally used during pregnancy. There is a slight possibility, however, that birth-control pills and vaginal spermicides may increase the chance of birth defects when used early in pregnancy. While the risk is very low, it is better not to get pregnant while using such contraceptives. If you find out that you are pregnant while using the pill, a diaphragm, or a spermicidal agent, stop the contraceptive right away.

Getting pregnant with an IUD in the uterus, however, is definitely dangerous. Half of the apparently normal pregnancies with an IUD in place end in miscarriage, and more end in premature delivery. If you miss a menstrual period or have an unusually light flow while using an IUD, you should consult your health-care provider within a week or two. Having the IUD removed early in pregnancy doubles the chance of a successful pregnancy—from about 40 percent to 80 percent.

An IUD can pose a particular danger. Nearly 15 percent of pregnancies with an IUD in place occur in the fallopian tube rather than the uterus. This situation is referred to as a tubal pregnancy. It is often difficult to detect and always requires surgery. The fallopian tube is too thin and narrow to support a growing fetus; as a consequence, tubal pregnancy leads to severe internal bleeding, usually during the second or third month after the last menstrual period. Severe lower abdominal pain results,and rapid surgical removal of the tube is the only treatment available.

If You Have Trouble Getting Pregnant

As we said earlier, after most couples decide to have a child, pregnancy follows within a year. For 10 to 15 percent of couples, however, pregnancy does not come easily. If you are having difficulty conceiving, there are certain steps you should go through.

First, you should review the facts about the timing of sexual intercourse and fertility. Ovulation (the release of an egg from the ovary) occurs approximately 14 days before the beginning of your next menstrual period, no matter how far apart your periods are. The egg (or ovum) is susceptible to fertilization for 18 to 24 hours after ovulation. Sperm are capable of fertilizing an ovum for up to 72 hours after being deposited in the vagina during sexual intercourse, and the amount of sperm ejaculated is larger if the man has not had intercourse for some time. The optimum timing, therefore, is to not have sex for several days and then to have intercourse just prior to ovulation, or approximately 15 days before your period is due to begin.

If you wish to find out when—and whether—you ovulate in a given cycle, you can do so by buying a basal body thermometer and recording your temperature every morning before getting out of bed. A basal body thermometer is designed to record small differences in body temperature. Your temperature rises about 1/2° F

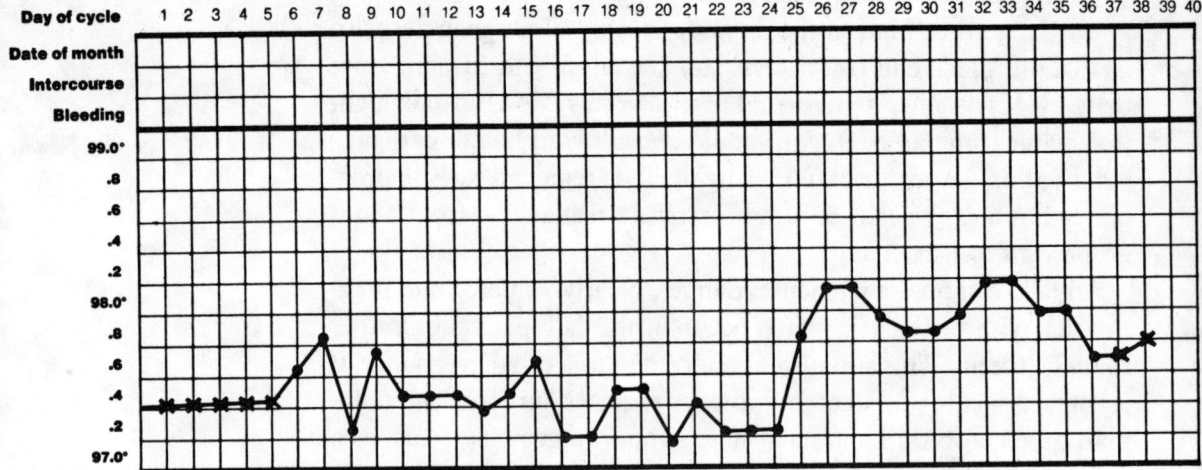

Fig. 1. Basal body temperature for one cycle. The woman who kept this recording had irregular menstrual periods. The rise in temperature indicates that she ovulated 24 days after her previous menstrual period began.

between six and 24 hours after you ovulate and remains at that higher level until just before your menstrual period begins. By keeping a chart of the sort shown in figure 1, you can record when in your cycle you ovulate.

Since the optimum time to have intercourse, if you are trying to get pregnant, is about a day *before* your temperature rises, the charting of your basal body temperature can only pinpoint in retrospect the best time to have intercourse. It does, however, provide useful general information about your cycles and fertility.

If you have been trying for about six months to get pregnant and have failed to conceive, we recommend that you contact your gynecologist or family physician to discuss possible solutions to the problem. At that time, you should buy a basal body thermometer and begin keeping a daily fertility chart. Use the chart on page 240 to record your daily temperature, your menstrual periods, and the times you have intercourse. Keeping a fertility chart will help you know when it is best to have intercourse as well as help you to identify the moment when you finally do get pregnant; the chart can also serve as a valuable record in the event that you need a formal medical evaluation for infertility.

If you have been trying to get pregnant for 12 months, paying attention to the timing of sexual intercourse, and are still unsuccessful, most physicians will recommend that you have a formal medical evaluation for infertility. In this context, the word "infertility" can mean just *difficulty* in getting pregnant, not inability, since medical treatment is frequently successful in bringing about a pregnancy. The medical evaluation of "infertile" couples can be quite complex and often extends over many months. Some identifiable reason for difficulty achieving pregnancy is found about 90 percent of the time, with 30 to 40 percent of difficulties related to the man and 40 to 50 percent to the woman. About half of the time when a couple undergoes evaluation for infertility, the woman will conceive during the treatment process. For those whose infertility appears to be confirmed, the physician will provide counseling about alternatives such as adoption.

Can a Couple Choose the Sex of Their Child?

Through the years, choosing the sex of an unborn child has been a topic of great interest and speculation. Certain methods of sex determination are based purely on folklore and often reflect prevailing sexual stereotypes—for example, the mother eating sweet foods to produce a girl, or the father having sex with his boots on to produce a boy. In recent decades, some intriguing research has linked the timing of intercourse with the sex of a baby. However, the value of that information for couples wanting a son or a daughter remains limited.

A couple wanting a boy can increase the chances of having one by not engaging in intercourse a few days before ovulation, and couples wanting a girl should refrain from intercourse until just after ovulation. Unfortunately, using this method decreases your overall chances of getting pregnant. Increasing the probability of having a boy from 50 to 65 percent might result in taking up to five years to get pregnant!

Several popular books and articles claim to provide a reliable method of choosing the sex of a child. The method is based on work by Dr. Landrum Shettles and includes directions about the timing of intercourse, the use of douches, positioning during intercourse, and advice on whether or not the woman should achieve orgasm. Shettles's work was based on artificial insemination data, however, and it is not surprising that scientific confirmation of his theories is not available.

To sum up, there is not yet a reliable method of predetermining the sex of a child. It is important, therefore, that couples value having a child of either sex. If you can do that, the rest can be left up to chance.

How to Find Out Whether You Are Pregnant

However much planning, serendipity, effort, or ease is involved in conceiving a child, most parents-to-be are anxious to confirm a pregnancy as soon as possible. For most women, missing a menstrual period is the first indication of pregnancy. But sometimes before a missed period is noticed a number of other changes in a woman's body can also signal pregnancy: breast tenderness, fatigue, and nausea, for example. As the uterus grows and presses on the bladder (three to six weeks after conception), many women notice a need to urinate frequently.

If you suspect you are pregnant, your next step should be a pregnancy test. There are two general kinds, both of which measure portions of a hormone called human chorionic gonadotropin (or HCG), which is made by the placenta. Its production doubles every two days in early pregnancy, peaking approximately eight weeks after conception and diminishing afterwards. *Urine pregnancy tests* measure HCG in the urine and are generally accurate by 10 to 14 days after a missed menstrual period. Blood or *serum* (since the test is done on that portion of the blood) *pregnancy tests* are more expensive but become positive earlier, often turning positive by the time of a missed menstrual period. They can be of particular value to women who are concerned about an unplanned pregnancy, or who wish to decide whether or not to use or continue contraceptives such as the pill. *Home pregnancy tests* measure HCG in urine and are generally quite reliable by four weeks after conception (two weeks after a missed menstrual period). Their cost ranges between $8 and $20.

Although pregnancy tests are basically quite accurate, they do occasionally provide misinformation. Combined with certain bodily signs, however, a positive pregnancy test should remove your doubts and allow you to begin planning for the months of pregnancy and beyond.

PART II

The First Three Months

CONCEPTION–13 WEEKS

Yes, pregnant! It is exciting to be pregnant, yet you may feel disappointed that you don't feel more vibrant, but still be patient if you can. Things will get easier later. Your whole metabolism is adjusting to the life growing inside you.

—Sheila Kitzinger, *The Birth Diary*

Pregnancy can be divided into three stages, each of which lasts about three months. These stages are referred to as trimesters. Each tends to have a certain feeling or flavor, although one slowly blends into the next. During each trimester, the parents-to-be find that they have a new set of priorities as well as new questions and concerns.

The first trimester is a time of rapid change. You and your partner are learning to adjust to the idea of pregnancy, and you may not always feel your best. These are months when you may often feel tired and nauseated. And it is understandable that you would have questions about the possibility of miscarriage, which is a common concern at this stage of pregnancy. During these months, too, you and your partner will need to think about various aspects of your relationship as a couple, especially your sexuality.

Now is the time when you will want to learn all you can about your pregnancy.

4 Choosing Your Health-Care Provider

No one specialist will suit every mother-to-be. The choice of a health-care provider is a highly personal one, and in most communities there are many good options available. Your choice is important enough to warrant investing some time and thought. If you haven't already made a decision with which you are completely comfortable, plan to shop around.

People Who Know How to Deliver a Baby

There are four kinds of specialists who are trained to provide prenatal care and to deliver babies.

Obstetricians have completed medical school and usually have spent four additional years of residency in obstetrics and gynecology. They are specialists in the treatment of diseases that can affect a woman's reproductive system, and they are, as a rule, well versed in the most advanced technology related to such treatment. A major portion of their training is surgical; they are the only specialists who handle high-risk pregnancies and who perform caesarean sections. To be certified by the Board of the American College of Obstetricians and Gynecologists, a physician must pass a rigorous examination of his or her qualifications.

Family physicians have completed medical school and have then spent three years of residency specializing in the relatively new field of family medicine. The approach of family medicine is to be concerned with the whole person, taking into account the patient's family, work, and community. Family physicians are involved in the treatment of people from pregnancy and birth through old age: they can provide prenatal care, deliver babies, and care for mother and baby after delivery. They often pay particular attention to getting to know the whole family. At most health-care centers, they are not the ones who perform caesarean sections or manage high-risk pregnancies; but they *are* trained in fetal monitoring and modern obstetrics.

Certified nurse-midwives hold an R.N. degree, and they must have had at least one additional year of clinical experience in maternity care and delivery before they are eligible to take the examination given by the American College of Nurse-Midwives. Though the laws regarding their qualifications vary from state to state, nurse-midwives are usually required to practice under the supervision of a physician. They are trained to work only with normal pregnancies, and they must refer any complication to a physician. Maternity centers and home birth centers are often run by nurse-midwives. They often spend more time with patients, both during office visits and labor, than a physician would.

Lay midwives receive their training by apprenticing themselves to another lay midwife and by studying on their own. They do not have professional training; nor have they taken an examination to certify their qualifications. In most states their practice is illegal. As more pregnant women choose to have their babies at home, there is more demand for the services of lay midwives; but because they lack formal certification, their competence is hard to judge. Many communities have highly skilled lay midwives.

In the end, your choice of a health-care provider may have less to do with the provider's title or speciality than with his or her philosophy, approach to childbirth, and reputation in the community—and whether you like him or her as an individual. Do shop around, either in person or by phone. The checklist on page 241 can be used as a guide as you search for the specialist who will best serve your needs.

Where to Give Birth

Where your baby is born will be determined in large part by your choice of a health-care provider. Most physicians and nurse-midwives deliver babies only in hospitals or birthing centers; but there are exceptions to this rule. Lay midwives usually deliver babies in homes or birthing centers.

Hospitals handle the vast majority of births in the United States.

However, depending on your health-care provider, the hospital, and any complications during your pregnancy or labor, the setting in which you give birth may vary. Discuss the options available to you with your health-care provider, and tour the labor and delivery room or, if there is one, the home-style delivery room in the hospital. At a teaching hospital, which is typically part of a large medical center, some of the staff will be resident physicians in training, who are called house staff. You may be asked to allow house staff to participate in your care while you are in the hospital. You may, of course, decline.

Birthing centers are places that are set up to provide a more natural, home-like childbirth environment. They tend to be located close to or within hospitals so that a rapid transfer to special care can be made if a complication arises. Most birthing centers are not very different from *home-style delivery areas* in hospitals, which have been developed in response to consumer interest in natural childbirth. Birthing centers tend to be small, with a staff that is accustomed to working closely together. The doctors and nurses at such centers often appear to be more concerned about the individual than may seem to be the case in the labor department of a hospital.

Home birth is extremely controversial. A number of studies indicate that patients at low risk for complications who deliver at home do just as well as similar patients who deliver in the hospital. In fact, several studies have suggested that women who deliver at home are subjected to fewer medical procedures and have fewer complications.

On the other hand, about a third of obstetric complications occur in so-called low-risk individuals. Because of their fear of unexpected complications, most physicians oppose home birth. However, some physicians and midwives do assist with delivery at the patient's home.

If you are thinking about home birth, we recommend that you explore that option carefully. To begin with, find out whether you are at risk for complications during your pregnancy, which would make home delivery less safe. If you wish to give birth at home, do *not* try to do so without experienced help. In particular, inquire about the professional reputation of the health-care provider whom you wish to have assist with your home birth, and make sure that there is adequate medical back-up readily available in case of an emergency.

Physician and Hospital Fees

When it comes to planning prenatal care, everyone is concerned about expense. Paying *more* does not necessarily mean you will get better care. Many public clinics offer excellent prenatal care. Nurse-midwives and lay midwives usually charge less for their services than physicians do. The information given here can help you plan your financial commitments over the next months.

Most clinics and health-care providers offer, for a set fee, a "package" covering all prenatal visits and a postpartum visit in the sixth week after delivery. Routine prenatal laboratory tests may be billed separately or may also be covered in the prenatal package. Tests that are not routine, including Alpha Fetal Protein (AFP), ultrasound, and amniocentesis, are usually billed separately.

You will be charged a set fee if you have a normal delivery. If you require a caesarean section, however, there will be an additional charge.

Hospital fees for the mother include the following items:

- **room and board**
- **labor room**
- **laboratory**
- **delivery room**
- **pharmacy**

For the new baby, there is a physician's fee for inpatient neonatal care and a fee for circumcision (if you choose it).

Hospital fees for the new baby include the following services:

- **nursery** (per day)
- **pharmacy**
- **laboratory**

At your first prenatal visit, you should discuss with your health-care provider, a nurse, or the clinic's business manager the type of fees involved, the amount, and what arrangements there are for payment. You should have a clear understanding of the charges. Your insurance policy lists the services your insurance company covers and the amounts your policy will provide for various expenses. If you have questions about your policy, the company will answer them for you. Usually the health-care provider will bill the insurance company directly.

5 Prenatal Care

esearch studies have shown over and over again that women who come in early and regularly for prenatal visits have fewer complications and healthier babies than women who do not have regular prenatal care or who wait until late in pregnancy to contact a health-care provider. We are not sure exactly why this is, but we do know that many procedures are routinely done by doctors and midwives to identify problems early. Discovering problems early in pregnancy results in earlier treatment, which will often prevent problems from becoming serious.

Visiting Your Health-Care Provider

Prenatal care is a team effort conducted by the providers and office staff of a health-care facility. There are four general goals related to your schedule of visits to the facility:

- *To check on the baby's growth and development.* This includes checking the size of your uterus and seeing whether it and the baby are growing normally. By listening to the heartbeat and asking about the baby's movements, your health-care providers will look for signs that development is proceeding normally.
- *To check up on your own health and adjustment to pregnancy.* The objective here is to anticipate and minimize possible complications in the pregnancy. Your health-care providers will routinely check on weight gain, look for signs of diabetes and kidney disease, and measure blood pressure.
- *To perform certain laboratory tests that should be done in all pregnancies.* These include a blood test for syphilis, screening for Rh disease, and other blood studies.
- *To provide information and answer questions.* Pregnancy brings about many changes in one's body and lifestyle, and these changes are different for each individual and her family. Also, plans have to be made for the

delivery and for adjusting to a new family member. Regular prenatal visits offer you an opportunity to talk about your concerns.

The routine schedule for prenatal visits is approximately once a month through the seventh month, every two weeks in the eighth month, and every week after that. Because it's important to get prenatal care started on the right footing, your first prenatal visit should be made as soon as you are reasonably certain that you are pregnant.

What Happens During a Prenatal Visit?

Most prenatal visits follow a set routine.

First, you are weighed. No one is trying to embarrass you— weight gain is a good indication of how well the pregnancy is progressing and whether you are eating enough. Low weight gain during the prenatal period is associated with a number of complications of pregnancy, including low-birth-weight babies and premature labor. How much you should gain depends in part on whether you were overweight or underweight before you became pregnant. A woman of average weight should gain somewhere between twenty and thirty pounds. Women who were underweight before pregnancy should gain at least thirty pounds, and those who were overweight should typically restrict weight gain to between fifteen and twenty pounds.

Next, you are asked to provide a urine specimen, which the nurse then checks for sugar and protein. Women who develop diabetes during pregnancy usually have sugar in their urine. Protein in the urine may be a sign of preeclampsia, an uncommon and potentially serious complication of pregnancy that leads to high blood pressure and kidney problems.

Then, you are taken to an examining room. There the nurse asks you some questions about the pregnancy and checks your blood pressure. It's important to check blood pressure during every visit because it sometimes goes up as pregnancy advances. Blood pressure that goes up abnormally may be a sign of preeclampsia, but it may just indicate a tendency to have high blood pressure. Whatever the cause, high blood pressure in pregnancy must be watched closely.

The physician or midwife always checks the size of the uterus, listens to the heartbeat, and asks questions about the pregnancy. The uterus should grow at a predictable rate. If the uterus is growing too slowly, that could mean the baby's development has been in some way impeded. If the uterus is growing too rapidly, your health-care provider will look for a cause, such as twins or an un-usually large amount of amniotic fluid. How big you look is not a good indication of how the baby or the uterus is growing, and that's why we measure the uterus with a tape. In fact, the amount your abdomen sticks out has more to do with muscle tone in the abdominal wall, and whether you've had babies in the past, than with how your baby is growing.

By ten to twelve weeks after your last menstrual period, your baby's heartbeat can usually be heard with a special stethoscope called a doptone. The doptone sends out a weak ultrasonic signal and records the reflection of that signal from moving objects. What your health-care provider hears is a reflection from moving blood or from movements of the baby's heart, rather than the heartbeat itself. That is why the sound of the doptone is often more like a "whoosh" than a "thump."

By about 18 to 20 weeks after your last menstrual period, your health-care provider can usually hear the baby's heart with a feto-scope, which is a type of stethoscope that fits tightly over the lis-tener's head. A baby's heart beats faster than an adult's, and the normal rate is anywhere between about 120 and 160 beats per minute. There's an old saying that a fast heartbeat is more likely to be a girl and that a slow heartbeat is most likely a boy. Don't count on it.

It is important that you let your health-care provider know about any sudden changes in the way you feel. Some health condi-tions need to be reported right away. In the box on the next page, you will find a list of conditions that could have a serious effect on your pregnancy.

Laboratory Tests

Certain laboratory tests are commonly performed during prenatal care, and many of them are done at the time of the first prenatal visit. Some are repeated several times during the prenatal period. Others are not needed by all women but are administered quite frequently anyway. On page 242, there is a checklist on which you can keep a record of your own lab tests.

Hematocrit (Blood Count). This measures the percentage of red cells in your blood. Red cells carry oxygen to the baby and are an indication of nutritional health (in particular, whether you've been getting enough iron). A low blood count can make you feel tired

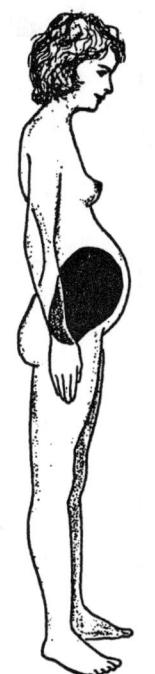

Poor muscle tone

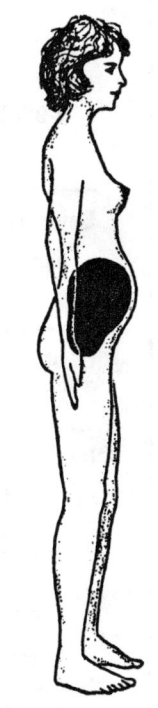

Good muscle tone

Fig. 2. How big you look is not a good indication of how the baby is growing.

31

Conditions That Should Be Reported to Your Health-Care Provider

Condition	Why your health-care provider needs to know
Vaginal bleeding	
up to 36 weeks, any bleeding of more than a few drops	*early in pregnancy:* threatened miscarriage
over 36 weeks, any bleeding of more than 2 tablespoons	*later in pregnancy:* possible bleeding from the placenta
Lower abdominal contractions, pressure, or cramps	
especially if occurring regularly 10 minutes apart or more frequently and not relieved by rest and fluids	*early in pregnancy:* signs of impending miscarriage, especially if accompanied by bleeding *later in pregnancy:* possible signs of premature labor
Vomiting	
lasting more than 24 hours, especially if it prevents you from keeping any liquids down	you may become dehydrated, if you don't seek treatment
Burning or pain with urination	
especially if you also have lower back pain	you may have a bladder or kidney infection
Rapid weight gain, with swelling of legs, face, and hands	
more than 3 lbs. per week	you may have preeclampsia
Severe headaches and spots in front of eyes	
alone or in combination with weight gain, swelling, and high blood pressure	you may have preeclampsia
Gush or leakage of fluid from vagina ("water breaking")	labor may be imminent; the baby needs to be checked
If you don't feel your baby move for one day	
first, drink 8 oz. of orange juice or other high-sugar drink, then lie down on your side for an hour and count the baby's movements; if you count three or fewer, call your health-care provider	the baby's health may be declining
Signs of labor	
"bloody show," uterine contractions, or water breaks	to review your health status and discuss your care during labor (talk with your health-care provider about labor at the start of the third trimester)

and can keep the baby from growing well. During pregnancy, the hematocrit is normally between 33 and 40 percent. It is generally checked at least twice, once at the first visit and once at the beginning of the third trimester.

Blood Type and Antibody Screen. There are two major parts to your blood type, ABO and Rh. Your blood type is reported as a letter and a sign, with the letter(s) (A, B, AB, or O) representing your ABO type and the sign (+ or −) representing your Rh type. These are important for your health-care provider to know, because if the father is of a different blood type, there is a possibility that your body will make substances (called antibodies) that can cause anemia in the baby prior to birth. This anemia problem is potentially most severe when an Rh-negative mother has an Rh-positive baby. It used to cause serious difficulties during some pregnancies, but now it can almost always be prevented by proper testing and treatment. This testing involves checking the blood type early in pregnancy. Rh-negative women (some physicians test all women) will be checked several times in pregnancy for the formation of antibodies.

Rubella Titer. This is a blood test that measures whether or not you are immune to rubella (German measles). While mild in the mother, rubella can cause serious deformities in a fetus if the disease is contracted during the first trimester. Most women are immune because they either had rubella as children or received a rubella vaccination in the past. The rubella titer is reported as a ratio, with a ratio of 1:8 or greater indicating adequate immunity. If your rubella titer is less than 1:8 (for example, 1:2), there is nothing we can do during this pregnancy to protect you, but you should receive an immunization shot after your baby is born.

Blood Test for Syphilis. This test looks for unsuspected syphilis infection, which can cause severe birth defects and illness in babies.

Gonorrhea Culture. Gonorrhea can cause blindness in newborns. A woman can carry the gonorrhea bacterium on her cervix without being aware of it; thus many physicians culture for gonorrhea at one of the regular prenatal visits.

Pap Test. This well-known test looks for early signs of cervical cancer. It should be done routinely whether a woman is pregnant or not, and we generally take the opportunity at a prenatal visit to perform a Pap test. The test itself involves mildly scraping the surface layer of cells from the cervix during a pelvic examination and preserving the cells on a glass slide. The slide is later examined under a microscope for signs of cancer or of conditions that could develop into cancer.

Urine Culture. Some women who feel perfectly healthy have bacteria in their urine. In pregnancy this condition should be treated because it is associated with the development of kidney infections, premature labor, and poor growth of the fetus. The urine culture, which tests for unsuspected bacteria in the urine, requires you to collect the cleanest urine specimen you can. A laboratory technician will then incubate a portion of the sample to see whether bacteria are present.

Alpha Fetal Protein Screening Test. This optional test involves drawing a blood sample between 15 and 18 weeks after a woman's last menstrual period. It measures a chemical that is normally produced by the growing fetus and not by adults. The amount of this chemical in the mother's bloodstream will be particularly high if she is carrying a fetus with certain very serious malformations involving the brain, spinal column, or intestinal tract. If the test is positive, a repeat test should be done. If the second test is also positive, ultrasound and possibly amniocentesis will be recommended to determine whether the baby is abnormal.

In more than half the instances when an alpha fetal protein test is positive, there is in fact no problem with the baby. Either the pregnancy is farther advanced than the health-care provider thought, the mother is carrying twins, or no cause can be found for the abnormal result. However, this test can detect conditions that are often fatal to babies. Many couples request alpha fetal protein screening in order to prepare themselves emotionally for the death or malformation of their baby; they may then consider having a therapeutic abortion.

Ultrasound. This common test is useful in estimating how far along a pregnancy is, detecting twins, looking for abnormalities such as hydrocephalus (head swelling caused by too much fluid inside the brain), and finding out where in the uterus the placenta is attached. Mild ultrasonic signals are sent out, reflected off parts of the baby, and picked up by a microphone. So far as we know, it is totally safe.

Before the test is administered, you are asked to drink lots of water because a full bladder will generate a better sonogram. After you lie down on your back on an examining table, your stomach is coated with mineral oil, which acts as a conductor for the ultra-sonic signals. A technician then moves a microphone back and forth over your abdomen, and the reflected waves produce a picture on a screen. It takes some experience to recognize arms, legs, placenta, head, heart, and so on, but usually the technician is glad to point these out for you. The test is painless except for the discomfort of having a full bladder. Because the test is somewhat expensive (about $50-$150) and has a theoretical risk (as any test does), it is not recommended routinely.

Amniocentesis. If a woman is at high risk for having a baby with certain diseases, her health-care provider will probably recommend amniocentesis. The test is particularly for women over 37, whose babies are more likely to have Down's Syndrome, and for those who have previously given birth to children with certain hereditary crippling diseases. A technician passes a needle through the woman's abdomen into the uterus and withdraws a small amount of amniotic fluid. The fluid is then analyzed for specific signs of disease.

Amniocentesis is usually performed when a woman is in her sixteenth week of pregnancy. The patient is placed on a bed or stretcher, her stomach is numbed, and she will probably feel a little deep discomfort or cramping. Ultrasound is used to locate the amniotic fluid and to ensure that the needle avoids the placenta and fetus. There is a small risk (less than one in two hundred) of causing miscarriage. Otherwise, amniocentesis is relatively risk-free. For women who have this test, the biggest problem is generally the anxiety of awaiting the results, which often are not available for several weeks.

Risk Assessment

For doctors, midwives, nurses, and other health-care professionals, the basic goal of prenatal care is to increase the chances that a healthy baby will be born to a healthy mother. We provide information, perform screening tests, and treat medical problems with that simple goal in mind. When making decisions during pregnancy, your chance of complications ("risk") must be taken into account. For example, the degree of risk needs to be considered in deciding whether you should plan a vacation, or in determining how soon you should go to the hospital after labor begins.

Estimating the likelihood of complications is a difficult task. Because each pregnancy is unique, there is no foolproof method of anticipating problems. However, we can apply information from thousands of pregnancies to make an estimate of risk. As you continue with prenatal care, your health-care provider will be able to make an assessment of possible problems in your pregnancy.

On pages 243–44, you will find a Risk Assessment Worksheet that will give you an idea of how the chance of complications is estimated. By mid-pregnancy, you should have enough information to make use of our scoring system. When labor begins, you can go on to the next step in assessing the chance of complications. Be reassured, however, that even if your score indicates a high degree of risk, the chances remain good that you will have a healthy baby.

Your Estimated Due Date

An important factor in prenatal care is an accurate estimate of your due date, particularly if you develop a complication during pregnancy. For example, the treatment of ruptured membranes (a "leaking bag of waters") and many other prenatal problems will differ depending on how far along the pregnancy is.

Not all pregnancies take the same number of days to mature; there may be a difference of as much as a couple of weeks. Our estimate of when your baby is "due" is therefore based on averages and may be off by as much as a week or two. Only about 5 percent of women actually deliver on their due date, but well over half deliver within 10 days of an accurately estimated due date.

On the average, pregnancies take 38 weeks after conception to mature. Since conception occurs at ovulation, which is about two weeks after the beginning of a menstrual period, the due date is commonly said to fall 40 weeks after the beginning of the last menstrual period.

Here's how to estimate your due date: from the date of your last menstrual period, count back three months and then add seven days. This date will be 40 weeks after your last menstrual period. For example, if your last menstrual period was April 17, count back three months to January 17 and add seven days: your due date is January 24.

If your periods are extremely irregular, or you are uncertain when you had your last period, you can use information about the progress of your pregnancy in your attempt to formulate an estimated due date. If you do know when your last period occurred, this information will be of help in confirming the estimated due date. For example, during the first trimester, a doctor or nurse-midwife can judge from a pelvic examination about how many weeks you are pregnant because the uterus is growing at a relatively rapid rate. Ask your health-care provider how large your uterus appeared on your first prenatal visit and use this information to confirm or recalculate the date of your last menstrual period.

A second way to check on your estimated due date is by noting when you first feel the baby move. This generally occurs at about the eighteenth week in first pregnancies and at about the sixteenth week in subsequent pregnancies.

When a woman's due date is uncertain, which usually happens because of missing or conflicting information, physicians often request an ultrasound test. With this test, a technician can measure the diameter of the baby's head, which grows at a standard rate in almost all pregnancies. Ultrasound is most reliable for predicting a due date when it's performed in mid-pregnancy, between about the eighteenth and twenty-fifth weeks; the resulting estimate of the age of a pregnancy is usually off by no more than about ten days.

To estimate your own due date, you should use all the information available to you. Where there are inconsistencies, it is best to point these out to your health-care provider and ask his or her opinion.

Here are a few additional pointers that may be helpful in dating your pregnancy:

- Between about 16 and 36 weeks, the size of your uterus is about the same number in centimeters, when measured from the pubic bone, as you are weeks pregnant. (You can feel your pubic bone beneath your pubic hair.) Thus, at 26 weeks, the average uterus measures 26 centimeters. At each prenatal visit, you will notice that your uterus is measured.
- The heartbeat can be first heard with an ultrasonic stethoscope (doptone) at about 10 to 12 weeks.
- Black women frequently deliver a week or two earlier than white women.
- The women in some families tend to have pregnancies that are consistently a week or two longer or shorter than 40 weeks. If you are pregnant, ask your mother and sisters about their pregnancies to find out whether there is a consistent pattern in your family. Don't be surprised if you follow the same pattern.

The worksheet on page 245 will help you in calculating your own estimated due date.

6 Nutrition

aking sure that you have an excellent diet during pregnancy is one of the best ways you can protect the health of your baby. And the great thing about nutrition is that, for the most part, *you* can control it. *You* make the decisions every day about what you eat. It's best to be eating well before you become pregnant, but if you need to improve your diet, now is the time to start.

In this chapter, we provide you with information that will help you make your pregnancy diet a healthy one. After reading it, complete the Food Diary on pages 246–48, write down your goals on page 249, and begin your prenatal nutrition program.

Principles of Good Nutrition in Pregnancy

Medical research on nutrition, exercise, stress, and lifestyles has produced valuable information on how to maintain the best health throughout the stages of our lives, including pregnancy. This research has dispelled some old ideas and changed approaches that were accepted medical practice for a long time. In particular, diets that severely restricted calories and salt are now known to be dangerous. At one time, it was common practice to restrict the salt (or sodium) intake of pregnant women. One theory was that salt caused preeclampsia. Now, however, it is thought that pregnant women should salt food to taste, and that a restriction on salt intake may in fact be harmful. American diets usually contain more salt than necessary, so it's probably best to continue to use salt as you normally do. Restricting calories during pregnancy is dangerous because it makes it very difficult to get all the nutrients you need.

"Eating for two" may still be a good saying—but with a different meaning. Instead of simply eating a lot of food, you should strive to eat a balanced diet of body-building foods.

It is not really hard to have an excellent diet, once you understand the basics of good nutrition in pregnancy.

Here are the most important things to remember:

- Using our list of the basic four food groups (page 40) as your guide, eat a wide variety of foods every day, emphasizing fresh fruits and vegetables, whole grains, lowfat dairy products, and high-quality protein foods.
- Limit your intake of sugars, refined and processed foods, and foods that contain a lot of additives and preservatives.
- Salt your food to taste.
- Drink whenever you are thirsty. Water, lowfat milk, and vegetable and fruit juices are especially good for you.
- Use supplements for calcium, fluoride, iron, and folic acid as prescribed by your health-care provider.

"Nutrient density" is an important concept for you to know. It refers to the percentage of key nutrients in a food compared to the calories in that food. An example of nutrient-dense food is lowfat cottage cheese. One cup of lowfat cottage cheese contains 300 mg or 25 percent of your daily calcium requirement, and 31 grams or about 40 percent of your daily protein requirement, but only about 205 calories or about 9 percent of your daily caloric requirement. By contrast, chocolate cake is not nutrient-dense; it contains only three grams of protein (4 percent of your daily requirement) but has a whopping 350–400 calories, or about 15–20 percent of your daily caloric requirement.

The Basic Four Food Groups

You've probably heard about the basic four food groups most of your life. Using the "basic four" as a guide to eating during pregnancy is a good way to make sure that you are getting the variety as well as the quantity of foods you need each day. Since a variety of foods is necessary to provide the different nutrients your body needs, there is no one "perfect" food. Following the recommendations in the box on the next page and in Table 2 will ensure that you are getting a good diet.

The Basic Four Food Groups: Key to a Balanced Diet

Group One: Protein and Meat

Provides protein for your baby's growth, B vitamins, and iron

Sources: poultry, lean meat, fish, eggs, cheeses

You need two to three servings every day

Alternative protein combinations for vegetarians:
rice with beans, cheese, tofu, or milk
cornmeal with beans, cheese, tofu, or milk
beans with rice, bulgur, cornmeal, wheat, sesame seeds, or milk
whole-wheat bread or whole-wheat products such as macaroni with beans, cheese, peanut butter, tofu, or milk

Group Two: Vegetables and Fruits (raw, or cooked as little as possible)

Provides a wide variety of vitamins and minerals, especially vitamins C and A, as well as complex carbohydrates and fiber

You need four to six servings every day

Daily: one or two servings of foods rich in vitamin C, such as citrus fruits, tomatoes, tomato juice, green peppers, or potatoes
and
two servings of fresh green leafy vegetables, such as turnip greens, spinach, lettuce, broccoli, and brussels sprouts

Five to seven times a week: a deep orange or yellow vegetable such as carrots, sweet potatoes, or winter squash

Group Three: Grains

Provides B vitamins, iron, fiber, complex carbohydrates, phosphorus, zinc, and vitamin E

Sources: whole-grain breads, crackers and cereals, brown rice, corn meal products, pasta

You need four to five servings every day

Group Four: Dairy Products

Provides calcium, magnesium, phosphorus, riboflavin, vitamin D, and protein

Sources: milk (whole, skim, lowfat, dry), yogurt, cheese, cottage cheese, buttermilk, and soups and sauces made with milk

You need four servings every day, or the equivalent of one quart of milk

Vitamin and Mineral Supplements

The Food and Nutrition Board of the National Research Council sets our nation's standards for nutrition, which it calls the Recommended Dietary Allowances (RDAs). Table 2 shows the RDAs for pregnant women. Most of your RDAs can be met by following our dietary recommendations based on the basic four food groups. It is, however, very difficult to get the extra iron, folacin (folic acid), calcium, and zinc you need during pregnancy. That is why they are the most commonly prescribed prenatal vitamin and mineral supplements. We therefore recommend that you take a vitamin/mineral supplement (with zinc) as prescribed by your health-care provider. (Note: vitamins with 1 mg of folic acid require a prescription.)

Calcium is the one mineral that is not supplied in adequate amounts in the standard "prenatal vitamin." It is assumed that you will get your calcium from dairy products, since the four servings per day recommended in our diet plan meets the RDAs for calcium in pregnancy. A few women are unable to drink milk, however. If you cannot drink milk, speak with your health-care provider about calcium supplements.

Table 2. Recommended Dietary Allowances

Vitamin / mineral	19–22 yr	23+ yr	Extra amount to add if you are pregnant
Protein (g)	44	44	+ 30
Vitamin A (μg)	800	800	+ 200
Vitamin D (μg)	7.5	5	+ 5
Vitamin E (mg)	8	8	+ 2
Vitamin C (mg)	60	60	+ 20
Thiamine (mg)	1.1	1	+ 0.4
Riboflavin (mg)	1.3	1.2	+ 0.3
Niacin (mg)	14	13	+ 2
Vitamin B_6 (mg)	2	2	+ 0.6
Folacin (μg)	400	400	+ 400
Vitamin B_{12} (μg)	3	3	+ 1
Calcium (mg)	800	800	+ 400
Phosphorus (mg)	800	800	+ 400
Magnesium (mg)	300	300	+ 150
Iron (mg)	18	18	+ 30–60
Zinc (mg)	15	15	+ 5
Iodine (μg)	150	150	+ 25

Fluoride is now also thought to be beneficial. One study of 492 children whose mothers had been given 1 mg of fluoride daily during the last two trimesters of pregnancy showed that up to age 7½ these children had virtually no cavities. Talk to your health-care provider about whether he or she recommends fluoride.

Protein

American diets are generally very high in protein. During pregnancy your protein needs increase from 44 grams per day to 74 grams per day—an increase of about 60 percent. This extra protein is needed for, among other things, the growth of your breasts and uterus and the development and growth of the fetus and placenta. You should pay close attention to getting enough high-quality protein foods every day.

If you are a vegetarian and you eat dairy products and eggs, you can easily get enough high-quality protein. "Group One" in our list of the "basic four" includes alternative protein combinations that can be substituted for meat. If you follow our recommendations for your daily need of protein, you will be fine.

For vegetarians who do not include dairy products or eggs in their diets, it is more difficult to maintain protein requirements.

41

You might consider supplementing your diet with eggs and dairy products while you are pregnant. If you decide not to do so, consult a dietician or nutritionist. Aside from their lack of calcium and protein, strict vegetarian diets make it difficult to obtain vitamin B_{12}, which is necessary to prevent a type of anemia.

There has been a great deal of controversy over the role protein plays in preeclampsia. Some researchers believe that lack of protein during pregnancy is the cause of preeclampsia. The data are inconclusive, but we do know that protein needs increase during the prenatal period. It makes sense, then, to pay careful attention to getting enough.

Weight Gain

You might be wondering whether the pounds you'll be gaining will ever come off, and whether you should really be dieting now. It

---

High-Protein Milkshakes: A Tasty Way to Add Protein and Improve Weight Gain

Some women have difficulty gaining weight or getting enough protein during pregnancy. Consider having a high-protein milkshake as a mid-afternoon or evening snack. It's convenient, tasty, and nutritious. With imagination, you can create an endless variety of flavors.

Milkshake #1
Basic High-Protein

In a blender beat one raw egg into one cup of whole milk. Add 2 scoops of vanilla ice cream, 6 tablespoons of powdered nonfat dry milk, 1 tablespoon of honey, and a drop or two of vanilla. Blend briefly, and enjoy.

This shake contains approximately 550 calories and 26 grams of protein! For added flavor plus fiber and vitamin C, also use ½ cup of fresh or frozen strawberries, blueberries, melon, peaches, bananas, or cherries.

Milkshake #2
Nutritional Gold

In a blender, combine one raw egg, one cup of milk, 1½ cups of ice cubes, 9 tablespoons of powdered nonfat dry milk, 2 tablespoons of honey, ½ cup fresh fruit such as strawberries, 3 tablespoons of Brewer's yeast, and 2 tablespoons of wheat germ. Blend thoroughly, and enjoy.

This milkshake is a nutritional gold mine! It contains approximately 550 calories and 33 grams of protein, and it is loaded with minerals and vitamins. The wheat germ is nutritious and helps constipation, too. The Brewer's yeast is an excellent source of B vitamins and many minerals; it will cause gas unless you eat some daily, beginning with a teaspoon and gradually increasing the amount.

Table 3. Components of Weight Gain

Component	Average gain (lbs.)
Baby	7.5
Uterus	2
Placenta	1.5
Amniotic fluid	2
Increased maternal blood volume	3.5
Increased maternal breast mass	1.5
Stored fat and protein (maternal)	4
Increased maternal fluid retention	4
Total	26

used to be common practice for obstetricians to put their pregnant patients on low-calorie diets. Women were told not to gain more than 10 to 15 pounds during the nine months of pregnancy. They were warned that if they gained too much, they would have a very difficult time taking off the "extra" weight after the baby was born. Excess weight gain was also thought to cause preeclampsia and to produce heavy babies, who would have to be delivered by caesarean section.

We know now, without a doubt, that *it can be very dangerous to restrict your caloric intake below the necessary amount during pregnancy*. Restricting calories makes it almost impossible to get all of the necessary nutrients, including protein and calcium, that your body needs for the developing baby. Pregnancy is not the time to go on a diet. You'll have time for that, if you need it, after the baby is born.

There is a relationship between restricted diets during pregnancy and low-birth-weight babies. Low birth weight can put a baby at high risk for several problems, including respiratory and developmental difficulties. You need approximately 300 extra calories per day while you are pregnant to meet your body's increased energy requirements, and you should plan on gaining more than 20 pounds during pregnancy. During breastfeeding, 500 extra calories a day are required; even so, you will still lose weight. Table 3 shows the components of weight gain in pregnancy.

The American College of Obstetricians and Gynecologists recommends an average weight gain of 24 to 27 pounds during pregnancy. If you were underweight before you conceived, you may need to gain more. If you were overweight, you can gain less—if you are very careful to meet the dietary recommendations. It can't be emphasized too often that pregnancy is not the time to diet. The chart on page 250 shows the average weight gain in pregnancy. You can use it to chart your own weight gain and see how you compare.

Problems Associated with Nutrition and Diet

Morning sickness (which is not limited to morning) is a common complaint during the first trimester. Estimates are that from 50 to 75 percent of all women experience some degree of nausea during the first three months. Aside from the discomfort, morning sickness may worry you at a time when nutrition is so important. It is very rare, however, for women to have morning sickness so severely that their nutrition suffers. Do make sure that the foods you eat are nutrient-dense and high-quality, and remember that the nausea will usually lessen by the end of the third month. Try eating small, frequent meals instead of three large ones. The old advice to nibble crackers before you get out of bed is still sound and may help you considerably. A high-protein snack (such as cheese) before going to bed helps some women. Although morning sickness is temporary, do talk to your health-care provider if you are very uncomfortable, cannot keep liquids down, or need reassurance.

Indigestion, heartburn, and gas can bother you throughout the last two-thirds of your pregnancy. They are caused by a general slowing down of your digestive system. During the last couple of months, your growing uterus crowds your stomach so that it can't work efficiently; there simply isn't enough room for much food. You may not be able to completely avoid these annoying conditions, but there are several things you can do to minimize them. Be aware of foods that cause you discomfort, and avoid them if possible. Fried foods, cabbage, brussels sprouts, spicy foods, and onions are common culprits. Eating frequent small meals will give your stomach more room to work. Be aware of your posture: standing and sitting straight also gives your stomach room to work. If you are still bothered, ask your health-care provider about antacids—but don't take them without medical advice.

Constipation is a common complaint during the last half of pregnancy. The best way to avoid it is to eat a high-fiber diet, with plenty of whole grains, fresh fruits, and vegetables. Dried fruits, especially figs, prunes, and prune juice, are very helpful. You might try starting your day with a cereal that is not only high in fiber, but delicious and good for you: a mixture of wheat germ, cereal such as bran or bran flakes or other whole-wheat cereal, sunflower seeds, almonds or other nuts, and dried fruit such as raisins, figs, prunes, or dates. Drinking plenty of water each day helps. Exercise also keeps your system working better. Constipation is one of the primary causes of hemorrhoids, so preventing constipation can prevent hemorrhoids, too. Do not take laxatives without consulting your health-care provider first.

Food cravings, for anything from shrimp scampi to chocolate candy, are almost universal during pregnancy. No one knows why this happens, but if you have experienced this obsession you know how real it is. Cravings are usually not a problem unless you substitute a non-nutritious for a nutritious food too often. If you are aware of and practice good nutrition most of the time, there is no need to be concerned about occasional indulgences.

Pica is a craving for a non-food such as starch, clay, or dirt. It can be dangerous to mother and baby for several reasons: it substitutes a non-food item, devoid of nutrition, for more nutritious items; it can cause problems such as anemia and intestinal obstruction; and it may contribute to toxemia. If you experience pica, talk to your health-care provider immediately.

Maintaining a Good Diet While Working or Traveling

It takes extra planning to maintain good eating habits during your work week or while you are traveling on business or vacation. But it can be done. Here are a few tips:

● Always keep a nutritious snack like a piece of fruit, raw vegetables, raisins, peanuts, or whole-wheat crackers in your purse. Then, when you get hungry between meals or must delay eating for a while, you won't have to turn to the vending machine or hot-dog stand.

● When possible, carry your lunch to work. This not only saves money, but ensures a high-quality, nutrient-dense lunch.

● When you eat in restaurants, make wise choices. Even fast-food restaurants often have salad bars or baked potatoes. A salad of greens, raw vegetables, and a good portion of cottage cheese is an excellent choice. (Watch out for the potato salad, cole slaw, and macaroni, which are apt to be loaded with mayonnaise and even sugar.) When ordering from the menu, ask for whole-wheat breads. Milk is available almost everywhere.

● Instead of drinking soft drinks, keep a supply of individual-sized cans of fruit, tomato, and vegetable juices at hand.

● When you fly, you can order a vegetarian or fresh-fruit plate when you make your reservations. These meals are often more nutritious and more carefully prepared than standard airline food.

● At home, keep some supplies on hand for when you are too tired to do much cooking or just don't have the time. Some suggestions: canned beans and packages of taco shells for quick bean tacos; canned tuna packed in water; peanut butter; yogurt; cottage cheese, frozen whole-wheat crackers, breads, and rolls for sandwiches; all kinds of frozen vegetables; sesame and sunflower seeds to sprinkle on salads and vegetables; cabbage, carrots, apples, and citrus fruits, all of which keep for long periods of time under refrigeration; individual-sized cans of juices.

Eat Well: It Is Important

Food *is* expensive, but pregnancy is not the time to budget good nutrition out of your diet. Consider a high-quality diet an investment that you simply cannot afford *not* to make, and cut your budget elsewhere. You don't have to spend a fortune to eat well, but choosing the most nutritious food items is often more expensive. Remember that it is worth it! If you need help in affording a good diet, contact your Department of Social Services to see whether you are eligible for food stamps or the federal Women, Infants, and Children (WIC) assistance program.

During the nine months of pregnancy, you will need an extra 75,000 calories and about 7,500 more grams of protein. Making sure that you get the food you and your baby need is one of the most positive steps you can take to ensure a healthy baby.

7 The Benefits of Exercise

Pregnancy is not a disease, but it *is* a major stress on your body. A fit and strong body will be able to handle this stress more easily, and to recover more quickly, than a body that is not in good condition. No matter what your level of prepregnancy fitness was, there's a lot you can do to prepare for labor and delivery and to get in shape now.

The best way to start your pregnancy, of course, is to be in great shape from the beginning. If this is the case for you, congratulations! If not, you can do a lot between now and when your baby arrives. You are probably more conscious of your body now than ever before, and you want to do what's best for yourself and your baby. Like good nutrition, physical fitness has many benefits for *both* of you.

A vast amount of new information about exercise and its beneficial effects on our bodies has become known in recent years. We now know that the human body doesn't *wear* out, it *rusts* out. We understand the importance of staying active during pregnancy, and of resuming physical activity very soon after childbirth. This knowledge, however, is in a sense a rediscovery: most women over the years and around the world have not had the luxury of being inactive just because they were pregnant. In fact, western lifestyles have made us less and less conditioned for the extra stress that pregnancy puts on our bodies and for the hard labor of childbirth. Desk jobs, long hours of standing, modern transportation, and labor-saving devices have all changed the demands we put on our bodies. Most of us have to plan to incorporate exercise (and even relaxation) into our busy lives—but doing so is well worth the effort.

There are many benefits to be gained from a regular fitness program:

- Exercise will help you feel better physically and mentally. Regular exercise increases your overall sense of well-being, reduces fatigue, and makes you feel more energetic. Your heart, lungs, muscles, and blood vessels work the way they are supposed to. As your fitness improves, you also gain self-confidence and self-esteem.
- Exercise helps control your weight gain during pregnancy. Afterwards, it helps you lose weight and get your strength back.
- Regular exercise will prevent or alleviate many physical problems associated with pregnancy. You will have improved circulation, which helps prevent varicose veins and leg swelling. Your digestive system will work more efficiently, helping to control indigestion and constipation. Strong muscles will better support your back, helping prevent backache and fatigue.
- Physical fitness helps prepare you for labor and delivery. You will tire less easily, and will be generally stronger and more able to cope with labor.

Sports

Participating in sports can be an important part of your fitness and exercise program, as well as being fun and rewarding. Attitudes toward women participating in sports are changing rapidly. The 1984 Summer Olympics showed how women athletes have won increasing attention and respect. And there is greater acceptance of pregnant women remaining active in sports. Fortunately, there are very few activities that, if they are already an important part of your life, must be stopped because of pregnancy. Many women continue tennis, soccer, softball, swimming, running, biking, and dancing throughout their pregnancies.

If you are uncertain about the safety of a sport, use common sense and all the information you can gather. During the last months you may need to slow down, but chances are good you'll be able to continue to enjoy your sport throughout most of pregnancy.

Common Questions about Physical Fitness in Pregnancy

It's quite normal, and sensible, for you to have questions and concerns about exercise—especially strenuous exercise—during your pregnancy. Some of the most common questions are discussed here.

"If I don't regularly exercise, how intensively should I do so during pregnancy?" First of all, it is best not to try to increase your aerobic fitness *after* you become pregnant; it's risky for your baby. Abdominal and pelvic floor exercises are fine, and most women

will benefit from a walking program, along with a well-supervised prenatal exercise class. But if you were not actively exercising before pregnancy, put off the all-out program to "get in shape" until after your baby is born.

If you are in good shape, and are involved in a regular program of physical fitness, most likely you will be able to continue your activities throughout pregnancy.

"Who can give me straight answers about physical activity and pregnancy?" First, of course, there is your own health-care provider. But many health practitioners have little or no background in exercise physiology or sports medicine. If your health-care provider cannot give you the information you want, or has reservations about the exercise or sport you are involved with, get another medical opinion. Physical therapists and physicians specializing in sports medicine are good sources of advice, as are teachers of prenatal fitness classes.

"Won't I be risking injury or miscarriage by exercising?" Medical experts generally believe that there is no cause-and-effect relationship between even the most strenuous exercise and miscarriage. But that applies to women who were already active and fit before they became pregnant.

"Are there reasons not to exercise?" Unless you are under close supervision and have carefully considered your fitness program with your health-care provider, *do not* exercise if you have any of the following conditions: cervical incompetence, toxemia, placenta previa, high blood pressure, diabetes, or threatened miscarriage.

Rules for Safe Exercising during Pregnancy

● Your balance will be more difficult to maintain because of your shifting center of gravity. You'll need to compensate for this.

● Because of the added weight you are carrying, there is more stress on joints and muscles. Warm up and cool down for longer periods.

● Breathing properly during exercise is always important, but even more so during pregnancy. To be sure that an adequate supply of oxygen gets to your developing baby, be aware of messages your body is sending to you. If you feel much more tired than normal at a certain point in your routine or activity, slow down or stop and rest for a few minutes. The "talk test" is one way to tell whether you're getting enough oxygen: if you can carry on a normal conversation while you are exercising, you are probably okay.

● Before beginning any exercise program, consider what your level of fitness was before you were pregnant. Use good judgment and common sense, and seek expert advice for answer to your questions. Prenatal exercise classes are usually organized so that you can participate no matter what your level of fitness is. Walking is a great way to get exercise without the risks involved in more strenuous activity.

- In early pregnancy, nausea and tiredness may interfere with your ability to sustain an exercise program. Listen to your body: if you're tired, weak, or nauseated, it's not a good time to exercise. There will be plenty of days when you feel more up to it.

- During the first trimester, excessive body heat may cause birth defects. Be especially careful not to get overheated during these months.

- During the last weeks of pregnancy, a softening of your pelvic bones occurs in order to make room for the passage of the baby. Even walking can be uncomfortable for many women. Again, listen to your body when you are exercising. If you are uncomfortable or experience any pain, stop.

- Never exercise to the point of exhaustion.

- Always consult your health-care provider if you're worried that something may be wrong. Be aware of the signs of over-exertion (dizziness, chest pain, nausea). In hot weather, slow down. Be sure to drink plenty of fluids to replace what you lose from perspiring.

Now that we have discussed the benefits of exercise, as well as the precautions to be taken, we can turn to the specifics of a prenatal fitness program. In the next chapter, you will learn about the kinds of exercises that can help you most in preparing for pregnancy and labor.

8 Developing a Prenatal Fitness Program

A well-rounded fitness program for anyone, pregnant or not, incorporates four types of exercise:

- **stretching, warming up, and cooling down** exercises to keep muscles and joints resilient and flexible
- **calisthenics** to improve posture and strength
- **aerobic** exercise to improve cardiovascular and respiratory function, control weight, and increase one's sense of well-being
- **relaxation** to help one cope with stress and to provide peace of mind

In addition to those components, a prenatal fitness program includes special exercises to strengthen the pelvic floor and abdominal muscles.

In the following pages, we will guide you in developing your own program of stretching, special exercises, calisthenics, aerobics, and relaxation. Using the Fitness Diary on pages 251–52, you can then keep track of your weekly routine of prenatal exercises.

Before You Begin

Before you begin your personalized program, choose a place in your home that can serve as your "fitness center." It only needs to be a corner, but must be large enough to allow you to stretch out in all directions. If you plan to dance, jump rope, or run in place, you will need plenty of space. You will also need a floor mat or something comparable to make lying down and sitting exercises comfortable. A mirror is a nice addition—watching yourself is excellent feedback, and fun, too! Tack the Fitness Diary to a wall near where you exercise. You can then make sure you're doing the exercises correctly and check on your progress. You may also want to have a tape-deck close by. Depending on your mood and the kind of exercise you are doing, music can stimulate or soothe.

Designer work-out clothes are fun, but not necessary. At a time when you are likely to want to save money, they are costly. What you *do* need are comfortable clothes that won't restrict your movement or circulation. In cool weather, loose sweat pants and sweat shirts, with T-shirts layered under or over for added warmth, and athletic socks and sneakers or jogging shoes are just right. In hot weather, wear only what you must for comfort or modesty. Even if you have never needed a bra for support, you may find that your breasts are heavy and tender now, and will feel more comfortable while you are exercising if you wear a bra. A good sports or running bra can really make a difference and is well worth the price.

Finding time for a fitness program can be a problem. But if you are determined, you will find the time. The minimum time required for our program is about three hours a week. You may have to schedule very carefully to fit those three hours in, but you'll find it is well worth the effort. Even if your schedule is tight, do try to work in the minimum time. If you use either a Saturday or a Sunday, when you're more likely to have a flexible schedule, you only have to plan for two weekdays. Of course, if you can fit four or five sessions in per week, that's even better. You will note that the Kegel exercises don't require extra time. Also think of ways to get extra exercise, such as walking instead of riding or driving.

Stretching, Warming Up, and Cooling Down Exercises

Stretching your muscles before exercising prepares them and warms them up. It makes you less prone to injury or soreness. Stretching after exercise helps prevent muscle tightness and soreness. Stretching also has benefits of its own: it increases the flexibility and strength of your muscles and joints.

Yoga is an excellent way to stretch. In some communities, there are special prenatal yoga classes.

Even on those occasions when you don't plan for other exercise, try to do a little stretching. As a daily routine, it feels great!

Here are some stretches we recommend. Whenever you exercise, spend five to ten minutes stretching to warm up and cool down. Avoid bouncing or making abrupt movements—stretching should be gradual and gentle.

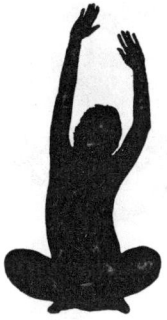 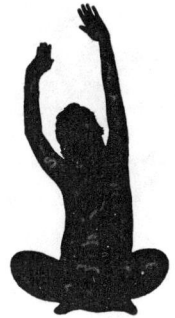

Fig. 3

Alternate Arm Stretches. You can sit or stand for these. With your arms outstretched over your head, reach for the sky, first with one arm, then the other. (These stretches will also improve your posture.)

Calf Stretching. With one foot in front of the other, and your palms against a wall, bend your front knee and gradually lean toward the wall. Repeat with your other leg. Don't stretch beyond your comfort level.

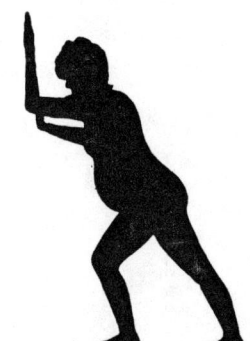

Fig. 4

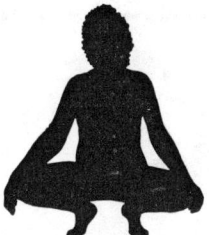 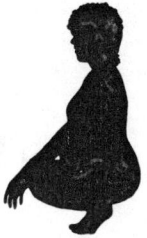

Fig. 5

Squatting. Do this as often as you feel like it. Squatting is good for easing lower back tension and for stretching calf muscles.

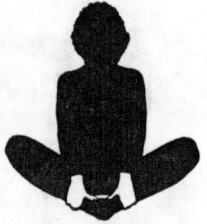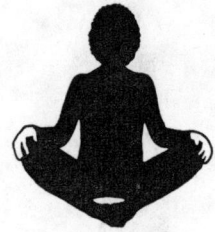

Fig. 6

Thigh Stretching. Sit on the floor with your heels together and pulled in toward your body as far as comfort allows. Slowly press your knees toward the floor; add a little pressure with your hands on your knees if you want.

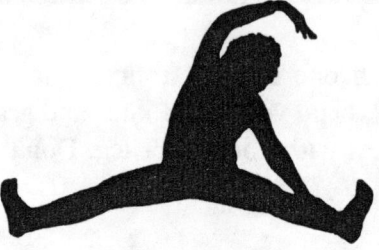

Fig. 7

Long Stretch. Sit on the floor with your legs spread. Stretch your right arm down your right leg toward your ankle. Bring your left arm over your head and *slowly* reach to your right. Repeat on the other side.

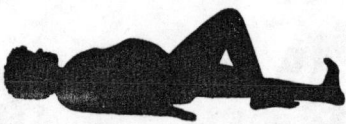

Fig. 8

Lying Down Stretch. Lie *flat* on the floor with your arms at your side. Bend your right leg and place your right foot flat on the floor. Flex your left foot up so that your toes point toward your face. Hold a few seconds. Repeat with your left leg bent.

Special Exercises for Prenatal Fitness

Pregnancy puts considerable strain on the pelvic floor and abdominal muscles (see figs. 9 and 10). Add the extra strain of sitting for hours, standing in one position, lack of strenuous exercise, and, possibly, being overweight, and you can see why our muscles are so unprepared for childbirth. The exercises described here will strengthen your pelvic floor and abdominal muscles for childbirth and should become a routine part of your daily life during pregnancy, and thereafter as well.

Well-toned pelvic floor muscles will stretch better during delivery and recover faster afterwards. Strong abdominal muscles will be called upon to help in delivery, and will help your stomach get back in shape more quickly. But there's another reason that makes these exercises even more crucial: preventing urinary incontinence (inability to control your bladder), prolapse (falling down) of the uterus, and other muscle-control problems associated with aging. Many people, including some physicians, believe these problems are an inevitable part of the aging process. Like many other notions about old age, this is just not true. Women who keep their pelvic floor and abdominal muscles strong with proper exercise are much less likely to have problems as they age.

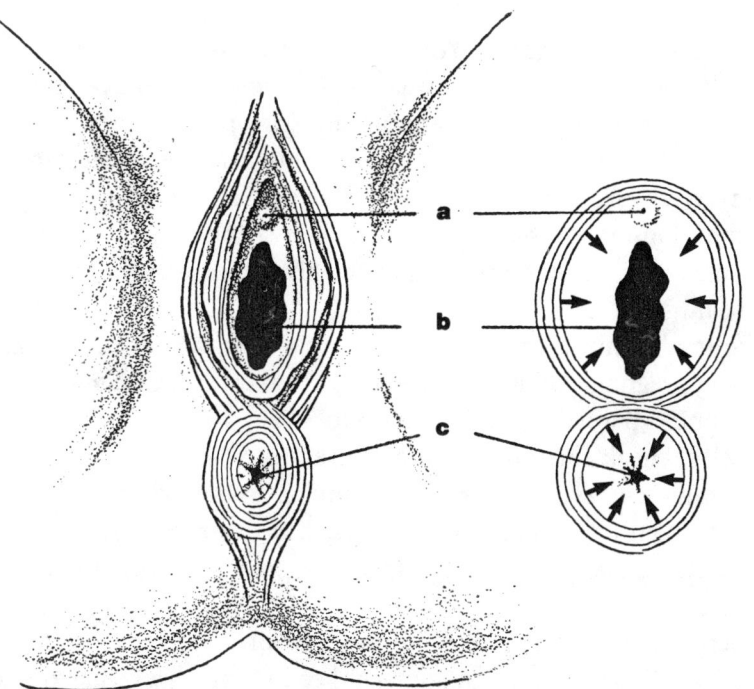

Fig. 9. The pelvic floor. The arrows show the muscles that are tightened during Kegel exercises: (a) urethra, (b) vagina, (c) anus.

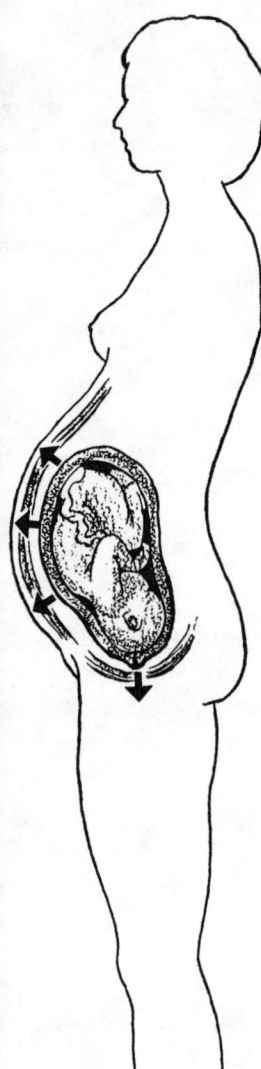

Fig. 10. The expanding uterus places a great deal of extra weight on the abdominal muscles.

Kegel Exercises. Exercises to strengthen the pelvic floor muscles are called Kegel exercises, after the obstetrician-gynecologist who developed them. Another name, coined by the physical therapist Elizabeth Noble, is "sexercises." These exercises strengthen the vaginal muscles, and strong vaginal muscles enable the vagina to grip the penis during intercourse, leading to increased sexual pleasure for both the woman and the man. In fact, many women say that the best time to practice Kegels is while making love: you have the benefit of a coach to give you feedback.

Kegels can be done anywhere, at any time. Try them while you are in a car, watching TV, reading, talking on the phone, waiting in line, and, of course, while making love. They can also be done in any position. Your legs should be slightly apart. Slowly tighten the muscles around your vagina and anus as you count to six. Then slowly relax to a count of four. Exercise for a minute at first and work up to five minutes at a time, several times a day. Breathe normally; resist the temptation to hold your breath as you count.

Here are two techniques to help you get the feel of the exercise: (1) Place your hand over your pubic bones. Imagine you are trying to contract your vaginal muscles as far up as your hand. (2) Try the exercise while you are urinating. If you can start and stop the flow of urine at will, you've got it.

Exercises to Strengthen Your Abdominal Muscles. Abdominal muscles are the other set of muscles requiring special exercises for childbirth preparation. Abdominal muscles play a crucial role in supporting your pelvis and back. In fact, as we've mentioned, many back problems can be prevented or alleviated by keeping your abdominal muscles strong. The increasing weight and stretch in your front throughout pregnancy will put lots of extra stress on these muscles.

Your abdominal muscles include two vertical bands (fig. 11). During pregnancy, these muscles may separate at the seam between the bands. Before doing exercises to strengthen your abdominal muscles, check for separation of these "recti" muscles (fig. 12). If your muscles have separated, you should do the exercise designed to prevent further separation. If not, you can safely go on to the more strenuous exercises designed to strengthen the abdominal muscles.

Here's how to check for separation: lie on your back (with your clothes off) and bend your knees, keeping your feet flat on the floor. If you can see a hollow (in early pregnancy) or a bulge (in late

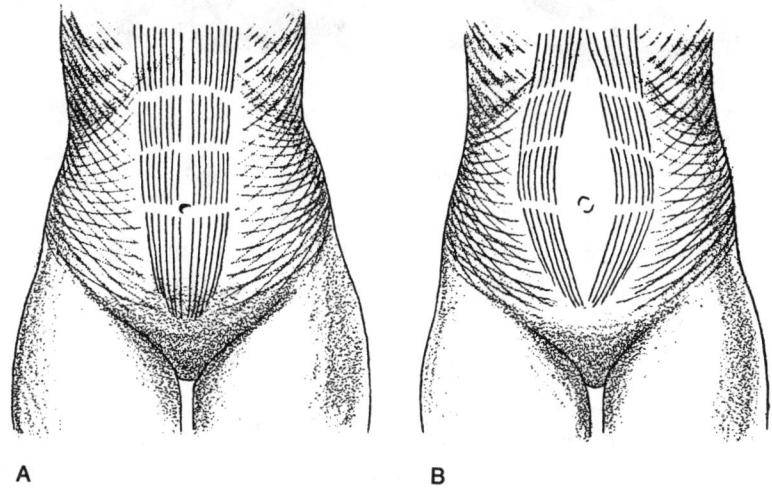

Fig. 11. Abdominal muscles. (A) The abdominal muscles act like a corset to hold in the abdomen. (B) Separation of the abdominal muscles.

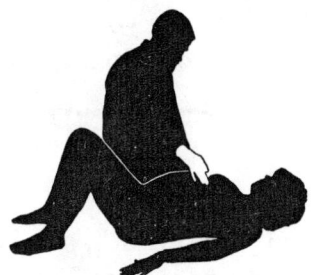

Fig. 12. Separation check.

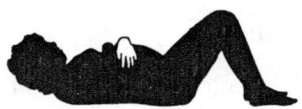

Fig. 13. Exercise for separated muscles.

pregnancy), your muscles are weak. Do the exercise for separated muscles to help prevent further separation.

Exercise for Separated Muscles. (See figure 13.) Lie on your back with your knees bent and your feet flat on the floor. Cross your hands and place them on your abdomen. Push the sides of your abdomen toward the center. Raise your head as you did in the separation check, but this time stop just before the point where you would see the hollow or bulge. Work up to doing this at least five times in a row, twice a day.

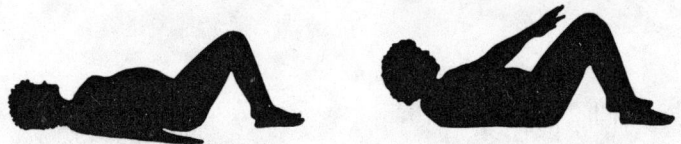

Fig. 14

Bent-Knee Sit-Ups. These are more strenuous exercises that will strengthen the muscular abdominal wall so that it will stretch less during pregnancy and be less flabby afterwards. Start the exercises as early as possible in pregnancy so that you can improve your strength level before your muscles start to stretch. The key to good abdominal exercises is to protect the lower back and to be in control of the leverage and resistance from gravity.

Lie on your back with your hands behind your head or at your sides. (If you need extra help, you can stretch your hands out in front of you.) Bend your knees and place your feet flat on the floor. Don't hold your feet down, as this puts the strain on your hips, not your abdominal muscles. The goal is to roll all the way up and to touch your elbows to your knees, but you may not be able to get that far at first. Start by rolling up as far as you can, then return to the original position. As your strength improves, you will be able to roll all the way up. If sit-ups are very difficult for you, start with just three or four a day, gradually working up to 15 to 20 a day.

Calisthenics

Calisthenics are exercises that can flatten your stomach, firm your leg and arm muscles, and add strength and tone all over. The word calisthenics comes from two Greek words: "kalos" for beautiful and "sthenos" for strength. For "beautiful strength," choose several of the following calisthenics. You may want to alternate the days you do calisthenics with the days you do aerobic exercise. Be sure to warm up and cool down before and after these exercises. Calisthenics should be done three to five times a week for 10 to 15 minutes a session.

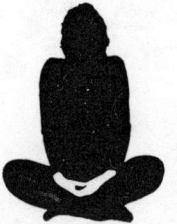

Shoulder Shrugs. Sit on the floor and raise your shoulders as high as you can while breathing in; breathe out, while letting your shoulders drop.

Fig. 15

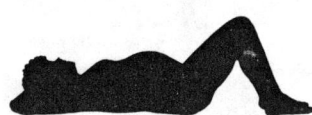

Fig. 16

Shoulder-blade Pinch. Lie flat on the floor with your hands behind your head and your elbows stretched out. Draw your shoulder blades together, forcing your spine off the floor a little. Hold a few seconds, then relax.

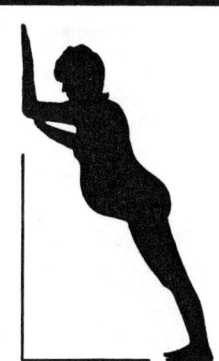

Push-Offs. Stand with your feet flat on the floor and your body straight, stretch your arms straight forward, and place your hands flat against the wall. Then lean forward by bending your arms, and push off by straightening them.

Fig. 17

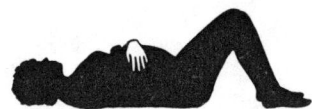

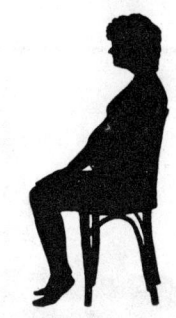

Pelvic Tilts. Pull your stomach muscles in, tighten your buttocks, and tuck your seat in. These can be done lying down or sitting in a chair.

Fig. 18

Standing Pelvic Tilts. Keeping your back flat against the wall and your feet about six to eight inches out from the base, tilt your pelvis by pulling in your abdominal muscles and squeezing your buttocks together.

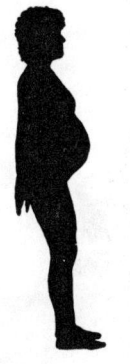

Fig. 19

59

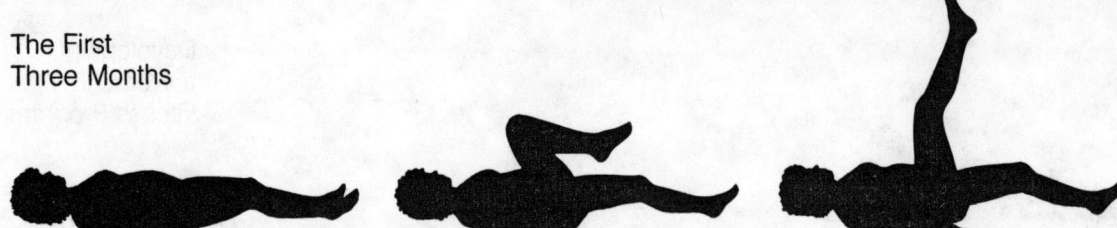

Fig. 20

Bent-Leg Hamstring Stretch. (1) Lie on your back with your arms by your side. (2) Bring your right knee toward your chest. (3) Straighten and extend your leg, flex your toes, then point them. (4) With your leg still straight, and toes pointed, slowly lower it to the floor. (5) Relax. (6) Repeat with your left leg.

Fig. 21

Pelvic Rock. Get on your hands and knees with your back *flat*. Tighten your abdominal muscles and pull them in and up toward your back. Tuck in your buttocks. Now relax and slowly let your back return to a flat position. Repeat.

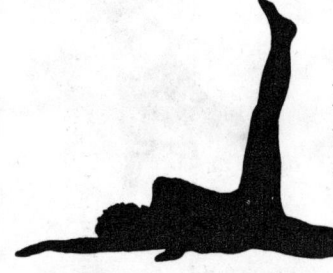

Leg Lifts (Lying Down). Lie on one side; raise and then lower your top leg. Relax, then repeat several times. Change to your other side.

Fig. 22

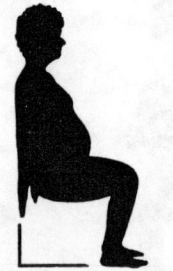

Imaginary Chair. With your back flat against a wall, pretend you are sitting in a chair. Hold this position for 30 seconds. Slide back up to a standing position, relax, then repeat.

Fig. 23

Side Leg Lifts. (1) Get on your hands and knees with your back flat and your face toward the floor. (2) Raise one knee to the side. (3) Straighten your leg. (4) Bend your leg and return to your original position. (5) Repeat with your other leg.

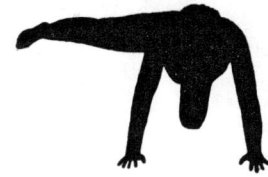

Fig. 24

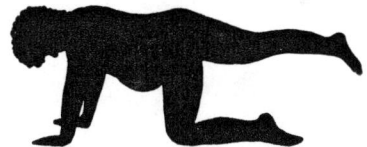

Fig. 25

Back Leg Lifts. Get on your hands and knees with your back flat. Straighten one leg back. Slowly raise and lower your right leg. Repeat with your other leg.

A Word about Posture

Maintaining good posture is more difficult during pregnancy, but good posture helps prevent backache and fatigue (fig. 26). Some of the calisthenics described above are particularly beneficial in their effect on your posture. Shoulder shrugs, the shoulder-blade pinch, push-offs, the three types of pelvic tilt, the bent-leg hamstring stretch, and the pelvic rock are all exercises that will strengthen the muscles supporting your spine.

Aerobics

Aerobic exercises must be sustained long enough to raise your heart rate to a certain point and to keep it up at that rate for at least 15 minutes. Running, walking, swimming, biking, and dancing are the most common forms of aerobic exercise. This type of exercise is the foundation of a well-rounded fitness program. Your cardiovascular (heart) and respiratory (breathing) systems benefit greatly. Done at least three times a week, aerobic exercises help you control your weight and improve your mental outlook.

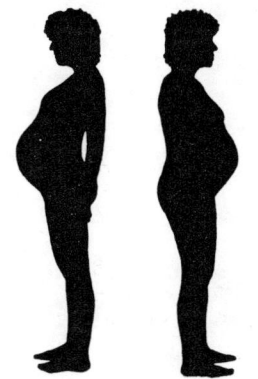

Fig. 26. Poor posture (*left*); good posture (*right*).

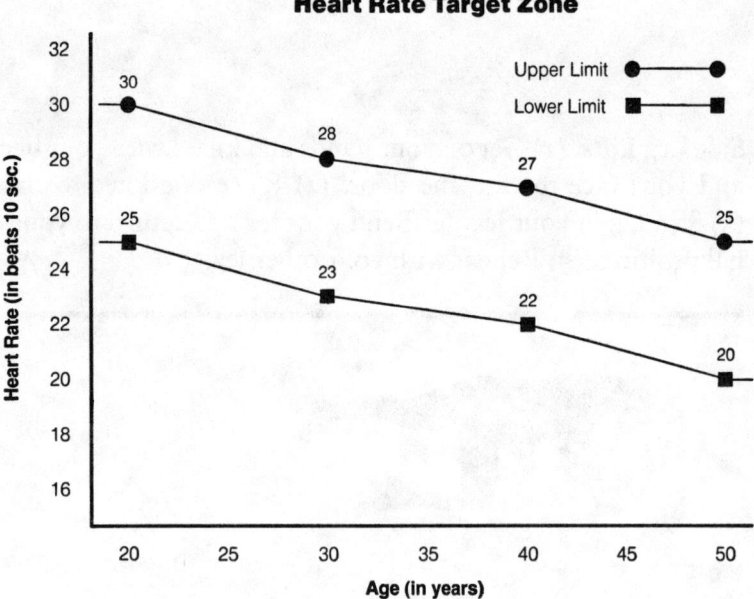

Heart Rate Target Zone

Fig. 27. Target heart rate chart. Use this chart to determine whether your pulse rate during exercise is right for your age. If you are in good shape you can aim for the upper pulse rate.

Once you have picked an aerobic exercise that suits you, determine your target heart rate by consulting the chart in figure 27. Then, after you warm up and have been exercising for a few minutes, take your pulse (see fig. 28). If it is in the target range, keep exercising at the same pace. The goal is to keep your heart rate at the same level for at least 15 minutes. Take your pulse again immediately after you stop exercising.

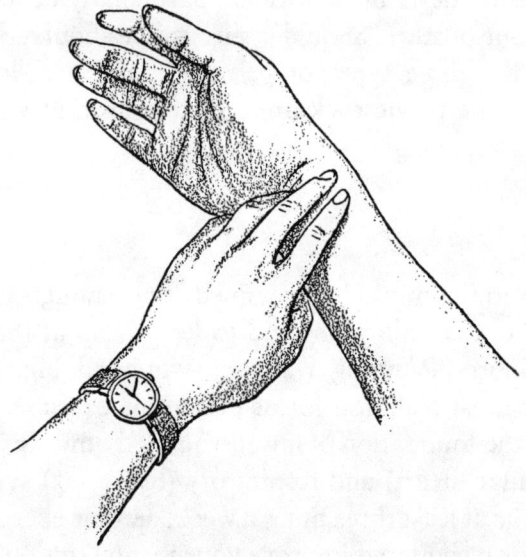

Fig. 28. How to take your pulse. With your index and middle fingers, softly feel for the pulse on the underside of your wrist. Count for 10 seconds, and multiply this number by six for your pulse rate. Always take your pulse *immediately* after you stop exercising because your heartbeat slows down right away.

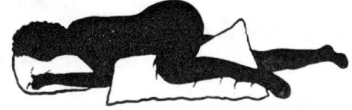

Fig. 29. A good position for relaxation.

Relaxation

Try to spend at least 10 minutes (more if possible) relaxing every day, using meditation, yoga, massage, or the exercise described here. Just lying down with soothing music, and breathing deeply and rhythmically, can be a wonderful way of unwinding. Figure 29 shows the recommended position for lying down.

Here is a basic tension-release exercise that is best practiced after an exercise session, when the muscles are slightly fatigued:

● Lie or sit in a supported position of total comfort. All parts of your body must be supported. The supporting surface should be firm; use cushions and pillows to accomodate your body curves and relieve all pressure points.
● Make sure all your joints are slightly bent.
● Keep your face expressionless and relaxed, and breathe quietly and effortlessly.
● Try gently checking your extremities to see whether they are relaxed. Gently raise one hand a little; if it is loose and heavy, it is relaxed. Then focus on your elbow, and proceed up to the shoulder area. Next check your thighs by rolling them in and out; rotate ankles, and check calves.

Massage is a useful aid. It will increase sensory awareness, improve circulation, and relieve stiffness and discomfort. It also feels wonderful! Have your partner work downwards from your head and neck, massaging your back anywhere that feels good to the touch. Slow, deep breathing also assists relaxation; each time you exhale, breathe out a little more tension.

Now, put your program together by filling in your Fitness Diary (pages 251–52). You don't have to do the same exercises every day, although you'll see improvement when you do. If you need a day off from your fitness program, by all means take it. Listen to your body; if something hurts, stop immediately. If you have questions, or doubts, ask your health-care provider. Above all, enjoy the increased well-being and energy you get from exercise—and know that you're doing something good for you and your baby!

RECOMMENDED RESOURCES

Noble, Elizabeth. *Essential Exercises for the Childbearing Year: A Guide to Health and Comfort Before and After Your Baby is Born*. Boston: Houghton Mifflin Company, 1982. This comprehensive guide to a preventive exercise program emphasizes the pelvic floor and abdominal wall muscles. Noble is a physical therapist and a pioneer in the field of fitness and pregnancy.

DeLyser, Femmy. *Jane Fonda's Workout Book for Pregnancy, Birth and Recovery*. New York: Simon and Schuster, 1982. Filled with excellent photographs and good information on fitness throughout pregnancy, birth, and recovery.

9 Environmental Hazards and Drugs

We live in a world full of chemicals, potentially harmful drugs, and other hazardous substances. In your job, at home, and even in your hobbies, you may deal with substances that could harm your developing baby. It is impossible to completely avoid all of them, but it would be foolish not to try. In the following pages, we discuss some of the harmful substances you may encounter in your daily life, and we provide information about ways to make your pregnancy as safe as possible.

For your peace of mind, it would be best to examine any potential exposure to environmental hazards *before* you become pregnant (see chapter 2). But if you are pregnant and feel you have been exposed to a dangerous substance, don't panic—consult your health-care provider or a public-health organization such as the March of Dimes (see page 71). The odds are heavily in favor of your having a healthy baby.

Lack of consumer information and knowledge about the dangers of prescription and over-the-counter drugs during pregnancy is alarming. As late as 1978, it was estimated that 82 percent of pregnant women were prescribed an average of four drugs (excluding vitamins and iron) per pregnancy, and that 65 percent of pregnant women took over-the-counter drugs.

Today, research and practical experience continue to confirm a statement made by the Consumers Union in 1972: "No chemical known to science has been proven to be entirely harmless for all pregnant women and their babies during all stages of pregnancy." Until the thalidomide tragedy in the early 1960s, doctors believed that most harmful drugs could not cross the placental barrier and thus could not endanger the developing fetus. Now we know that many stillbirths, miscarriages, and birth defects are caused by environmental agents and drug exposures. Though many birth defects can be attributed to hereditary and environmental factors, most abnormalities have no identifiable cause. So it is better to be overly cautious with drugs, chemicals, and environmental agents.

The Effects of Drugs during the Course of Pregnancy

No drug or toxin causes ill effects in all pregnancies. Whatever effect it does have depends on the dose, the length of exposure, and the stage of pregnancy at which the exposure has occurred. The higher the dose, the more likely it is to cause ill effects. Similarly, long exposures are more likely to be harmful than short ones.

During the course of a pregnancy, there are certain times when the developing infant is sensitive to toxic effects (see fig. 30). In the first two weeks or so after fertilization, the embryo has not yet begun to develop organs. At this early stage of pregnancy, toxins seem

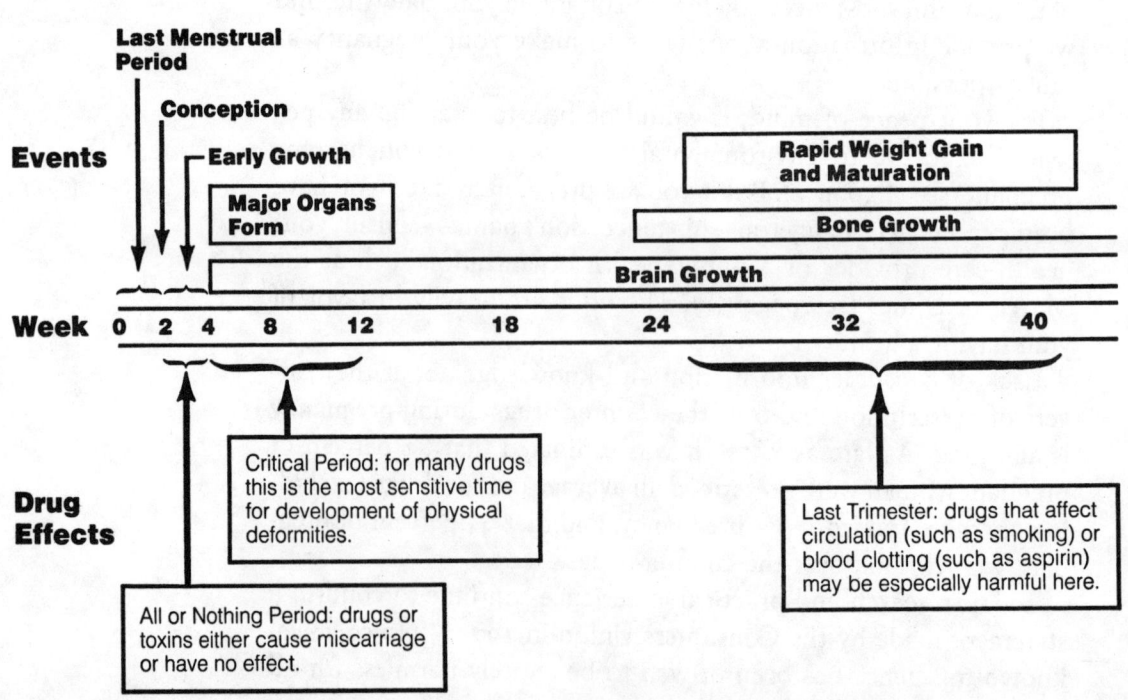

Fig. 30. The general timing of drug effects during pregnancy.

either to kill the embryo (causing miscarriage) or to have no lasting effects. The remainder of the first trimester, when the major organs are formed, is the time of greatest sensitivity to drugs: even small doses of harmful drugs can result in serious deformities. You should be most careful during early pregnancy to limit drug use and exposure to environmental toxins.

Later on, drugs and other hazards can still affect bone and central nervous system development, as well as the mother's circulation. During the second and third trimesters, fetal growth is rapid, and agents that interfere with growth, such as tobacco smoke, can be particularly harmful.

Prescription and Non-Prescription Drugs

If your health-care provider prescribes for you a drug, he or she should weigh the potential risks to the developing baby against the benefits for you. Some medical conditions have to be treated with a potentially harmful drug. In the case of less serious ailments, you should use a drug only if it seems quite safe for the fetus. Remember: we are not *absolutely* sure about any drug, but we have a good idea about the relative safety of most medications.

If you are regularly taking a prescription drug for a chronic condition such as seizures or asthma, it is probably less hazardous to continue use of the drug than to do without it. Some prescription drugs are safer than others, however. Be sure to discuss your use of medications with your health-care provider. The best time to do so is before you become pregnant; failing that, ask about the matter as soon as you start prenatal care.

If you are given a prescription, take it only as recommended, both for the length of time and in the amounts prescribed. If you are concerned about the drug's effects, talk to your health-care provider or look for information, using the resources mentioned in this book.

American women in general probably take more vitamins than they need. While moderate vitamin supplements are safe, large doses of many vitamins—particularly vitamins D, A, and K—can have damaging effects. Avoid taking a needless risk; stick to the recommended daily allowance of various vitamins and minerals (see table 2, page 41).

It is a good idea to keep a record of your prescriptions and of the over-the-counter drugs you have around the house for occasional use. On page 253, you will find worksheets on which you can make your list. Check your cabinets, purse, and bathroom to cover all possibilities. Are you surprised by the number of drugs on your lists? Most households have at least a dozen medicines around. While some may be safe during pregnancy, many are definitely risky.

Minor Health Problems

There may be times when you have a headache, a cold, or some other problem and are feeling miserable. Here are some guidelines for treating some minor health problems.

Morning Sickness. Many women can get by without any medicine by eating small meals often—even every hour. (See page 103 for further suggestions.) If you have severe nausea, consult your healthcare provider.

Headache. Both aspirin and acetaminophen (Tylenol, Datril) appear to be safe. Some doctors recommend acetaminophen in the first trimester, because aspirin is known to cause birth defects in animals. Most recommend avoiding aspirin in the last two months, because it can slow blood clotting, making you prone to excessive bleeding.

Constipation. High-fiber diets (see page 44), when combined with plenty of liquids, can usually prevent constipation. Prune juice is an effective laxative, if one is needed. Metamucil, a powder that is stirred into water or juice, is a safe, mild, effective over-the-counter drug.

Coughs and Colds. A vaporizer and throat lozenges may help. Decongestants such as nose drops or Sudafed are probably safe. Some physicians recommend that antihistamines not be used during the first trimester: their harm to humans has not been proven, but they do cause birth defects in animals.

Heartburn. A common problem in pregnancy, heartburn can usually be controlled by eating smaller meals and not lying down immediately after eating; resting with additional support for the upper part of the body can also be of help. Antacids such as Maalox, Mylanta, or Gelusil are probably safe. One study found a link between antacid use and birth defects, so they should be avoided during the first trimester.

Swelling. Your legs and hands may often swell, especially in the summer or when you have been standing for long periods of time. Lying down, particularly on the left side, is the recommended treatment. Avoid diuretics (water pills).

Itching. Some women are bothered by a lot of itching when pregnant. Witch hazel and calamine lotion are effective and safe. Hydrocortisone cream (0.5%, available without prescription) is safe but should be used for no longer than a few weeks. Benadryl (diphenhydramine) is probably safe, but requires a prescription.

Tobacco, Caffeine, Alcohol, and Marijuana

Cigarettes, alcoholic beverages, beverages containing caffeine, and marijuana fall into the category of social drugs. These, too, need to be considered in any record of the drugs to which you are exposed. Turn to the worksheet on page 254 and list all the social drugs that you use regularly or once in a while, as well as ones that you recently stopped using.

Tobacco. There is a direct association between smoking in pregnancy and low birth weight, miscarriages, and some birth defects. Smoking seems to be particularly harmful late in pregnancy. In the weeks just before birth, smoking more than a pack a day increases the risk of a baby's death by 35 percent; less than a pack increases the risk by 20 percent. Therefore, smoking as little as possible, and preferably not at all, is best for your baby's health. If your partner or friends smoke, ask them to do so where it does not affect the quality of the air you breathe. For smokers who wish to quit, a six-step program is outlined on page 255.

Alcohol. It is now clear that alcohol can have harmful effects on a growing fetus. Babies of heavy drinkers often display a pattern of physical and mental defects called *fetal alcohol syndrome*. No one knows how much alcohol is too much in pregnancy. For that reason, many doctors (including the U.S. Surgeon General) recommend that pregnant women *not drink at all*.

Caffeine. The hazards of coffee are not as clear-cut as the dangers posed by alcohol and tobacco, but animal studies have definitely linked *high* doses of caffeine with birth abnormalities, miscarriages, stillbirths, and premature labor. Since there is no clear evidence about caffeine consumption, avoid caffeine, or limit consumption to *less* than 250 mg of caffeine per day—three cups of coffee, four cans of cola, or six cups of tea.

Even less is known about decaffeinated coffee, which contains traces of potentially harmful chemicals that are left over from the usual decaffeination process. The water method of decaffeination uses no chemicals. Little or nothing is known about the effects of drinking herb teas.

Marijuana. Some doctors recommend that pregnant women not smoke marijuana since it is known to cause birth abnormalities in animals. Smoking marijuana has some of the effects associated with cigarette smoking, such as increasing the carbon monoxide content of red blood cells. Avoid using marijuana during pregnancy.

X-rays

Radiation exposure in high doses is known to cause cancer. There is little evidence, however, that radiation causes pregnancy-related problems or deformities in infants. The major risk related to x-ray exposure is probably the chance of contracting cancer, especially leukemia, several years later. For a radiation dose of 12 rads (20 times the average chest x-ray dose), the risk has been estimated at about one case of leukemia in 1,000 exposures.

Radiation exposure, therefore, does pose some risk during pregnancy. That risk is small enough, however, that x-rays should not be avoided if they are medically indicated. When an area other than your pelvis is being x-rayed—your hand, for example—proper lead shielding of your abdomen essentially eliminates any risk to the baby.

Ultrasound has replaced x-rays in many areas of medicine. It is often used to look at the baby and placenta. At present, there are no known ill effects to mother or baby from ultrasound.

It's easy to get frightened when you realize how many chemicals and drugs are around and how little is known about most of them. The best policy is to avoid exposure when you have a choice and to remain informed: then you know you are doing everything you can.

RECOMMENDED RESOURCES

American Lung Association. (Check your phone book for your local chapter.) Sponsors stop smoking groups and publishes free and inexpensive educational materials on smoking.

March of Dimes Birth Defects Foundation, 1275 Mamaroneck Avenue, White Plains, New York 10605. (Most communities have a local chapter.) Provides information on preventing birth defects.

10 Working and Pregnancy

It has been estimated that about 85 percent of working women will become pregnant at some point in their working lives. There are about a million pregnancies a year among working women, and more than half of the women who work during pregnancy return to work less than a year after delivery.

However, combining the role of worker with that of expectant or new mother can be complex. A working woman is likely to have special concerns related to pregnancy. Is my job safe? If not, what can I do? Can I lose a promotion or be fired for being pregnant? Will I need special consideration on the job because I am pregnant? How long into pregnancy can I work?

Those are increasingly common questions as more and more women with jobs and careers think about starting a family. Here we will provide you with information that can help you balance your desire to work with your desire for a healthy and satisfying pregnancy.

Recommendations for Working Women

Most health-care providers agree that if you wish to work throughout pregnancy you should do so—assuming that you are in good general health and the job itself poses no danger. Within that broad framework, you and your health-care provider should consider your age and reproductive history, as well as the nature of your job, including physical demands, potential hazards, stress, and time spent commuting. The accompanying box outlines the advice many physicians give working patients with normal pregnancies.

Recommendations for Working Women*

All Jobs

Try to:	Avoid:
Take frequent breaks	Exhaustion
Rest on left side at lunch hour	Discomfort
Stop working when fatigued	Extreme temperatures
Elevate legs periodically	Smoking areas
Take walks	Noxious odors and chemical fumes
Perform stretching exercises, especially for back and legs	Lifting more than 25 pounds

Jobs That Require a Lot of Standing or Walking

Try to:	Avoid:
Reduce activity; work part-time or at most in 8-hour shifts	Heavy lifting or pushing
Take naps or rest periods morning and afternoon	Excessive stair climbing
Empty bladder every 2 hours	Running
Stop or reduce work during the ninth month; wear support hose	In-flight airline work in final month

Jobs That Require Physical Exertion

Try to:	Avoid:
Use common sense	Heavy lifting and straining
Stop when short of breath	Prolonged standing
Empty bladder every 2 hours	Trauma to abdomen from heavy equipment
Get extra rest on weekends	Overtime
Exercise great caution around hazardous equipment, such as machinery with moving parts	
Stop work after 7th or 8th month or work part-time	

*Adapted from *Contemporary OB/GYN*, April 1982.

Some Practical Things to Consider

Sooner or later, you will have to make some important decisions regarding your job. These decisions, some of which are discussed below, should not be put off. Think about them early in your pregnancy, and explore your options.

- *When to tell your employer and coworkers about your pregnancy.* Once you decide to do it, be positive about it. Assume that your boss will be just as confident as you are that your work will not be hampered by your pregnancy. There may be annoying questions about *when* you plan to quit or whether you'll be coming back. These are questions you have to think about and answer sooner or later. Remember that you are not bound by your decisions; you have the right to change your mind. No one can predict for certain how you will feel physically or emotionally about continuing work until delivery, or when you will be ready to return to work after delivery.
- *Maternity leave and insurance coverage.* Before making a decision about these important issues, learn what options you and your partner have. Some employers provide paternity benefits, which allow fathers to participate more in early infant care. Working part-time at the end of your pregnancy and for a while when you return to work may also be an alternative. Practices vary widely; do explore your options. You may be surprised at how receptive your employer is to requests that are presented in a positive and well-thought-out manner.
- *Physical comfort on the job.* Unfortunately, most jobs are not geared to a pregnant worker's comfort. You will need rest periods and time to put your feet up. Frequent snacks can help keep your energy level up, as well as limit nausea. You'll have to make more frequent trips to the bathroom. All those things can probably be worked into your regular workday without causing much concern on the part of your employer or coworkers. If your job is inflexible, and you have done what you can to make some changes, you may face the difficult decision of whether to stop work early for health and comfort reasons.
- *Commuting.* This can be a hassle as well as a health problem. Women who have long commutes seem more likely to go into labor prematurely. In addition, commuting can be tiring. Changing your schedule so that you are not commuting at peak rush hours may help. Reducing your work hours is another possibility. Discuss the options with your health-care provider and your employer.
- *Tobacco smoke.* Pregnant women should not work in an environment that contains tobacco smoke. Ask your coworkers to refrain from smoking where it affects the quality of the air you breathe.

Assessing the Safety of Your Job

We are becoming increasingly aware of hazards in many industries, including reproductive hazards to potential mothers and fathers and to pregnant women. Too often, however, it is still up to the pregnant (or potentially pregnant) worker to learn about hazards in her job and to take steps to protect herself from exposure.

Ideally, you should assess your job and your partner's job for health hazards as soon as you begin planning to become pregnant. In this way, you may be able to prevent your exposure to hazards that may have an effect on a developing fetus but aren't necessarily harmful to an adult. At any rate, as soon as you suspect that you are pregnant, you should look at your job to determine if there are any hazards that could harm a developing fetus.

Table 4 lists occupational exposures that may have an effect upon pregnancy outcome. In particular, you should be aware of the following classes of hazards:

• *Chemical hazards.* The developing fetus can be easily harmed by chemicals, and some exposures can cause miscarriage or deformities. You should be especially aware of potential hazards if you work in one of these fields: textiles; pharmaceuticals; medicine (hospitals and operating rooms); the plastics industry; the petrochemical industry; jobs where you are exposed to automotive fumes; agriculture; dry cleaning; chemical plants or laboratories; crafts and any work that involve the use of solvents, dyes, pesticides, or heavy metals (lead, mercury, cadmium).

• *Environmental hazards.* Excessive heat, excessive noise, and high levels of mental stress should be avoided. Many office workers, especially those who work at video display terminals (VDTs), may have to deal with considerable stress. Recent studies have failed to find a relationship between VDTs and birth defects.

• *Infectious diseases.* Teachers, veterinarians, animal handlers, physicians, nurses, and hospital workers may be exposed to infectious agents. These include rubella virus, cytomegalovirus (salivary gland virus), herpes virus, toxoplasmosis, and syphilis.

• *Ionizing radiation.* Because developing babies are more susceptible to harm than adults, it is particularly important to minimize exposure to radiation. Women who work in fields that expose them to radiation (nuclear industry workers, nuclear medicine workers, x-ray technicians, dentists and dental assistants, and nurses who work with patients with radioactive inserts) should have their monitoring badges read monthly to ensure that their dose level has remained within the safety zone. The recommended x-ray dosage limit during pregnancy is 1.5 rem.

• *Physical hazards.* During the last trimester you are more prone to injury from physical labor such as pushing, lifting, climbing, or carrying heavy loads. You are also more prone to fatigue and muscle strain from sitting all day at a desk, machine, or VDT. Standing for long periods of time makes you more susceptible to varicose veins and fatigue; thus many physicians advise pregnant women to limit the number of hours they stand at work.

Table 4. Occupational Risks to Pregnancies

Exposure	Some occupations at risk
Heavy metals	
Lead	Battery-plant workers, smelter workers, foundry workers, painte demolition workers, plumbers, enamel workers, ceramic maker solderers, potters, pesticide workers, mechanics
Mercury and its compounds (*organic and inorganic*)	Disinfectant makers, seed handlers, wood preservers, fungicid makers, drug makers, dye makers, pesticide workers, tannery workers, amalgam makers, dentists, dental assistants
Cadmium	Battery makers, smelter workers, solderers, engravers, textile printers, welders, paint makers, metal workers, alloy makers, pesticide workers
Selenium	Photographic-chemical workers, glass makers, lab workers, pi ment makers, rubber makers
Tellerium and its compounds	Alloy makers, ceramic makers, glass makers, silverware make porcelain makers, rubber workers
Hypoxic agents	
Carbon monoxide	Bridge and tunnel toll-collectors, furnace workers, boiler-room workers, garage mechanics, miners, pulp and paper workers, workers
Anesthetic gases	
Halogenated gases (*e.g., halothane, methoxy-fluorane, nitrous oxide*)	Operating-room personnel (especially anesthetists and anesth siologists), dental and veterinary personnel
Pesticides	
Chlordecone	Pesticide workers, farmworkers
Chlorinated hydrocarbons (*e.g., chlordane & heptachlor*)	Termite exterminators and agricultural workers (especially cultivators and pickers of pineapples, strawberries, and Florid citrus fruits)
Captan, folpet, captatol, thiram	Pesticide workers, agricultural workers
Organic solvents and halogenated hydrocarbons	
Benzene	Laboratory workers, chemical workers, adhesive makers, detergent makers, furniture finishers, glue makers, lacquer work dye makers
Chloroprene	Rubber makers, latex makers
Ethylene dibromide (EDB)	Fumigant workers, termite controllers, fire-extinguisher maker wood reclaimers, resin makers

Table 4. *Continued*

Exposure	Some occupations at risk
Perchloroethylene (tetrachloroethylene)	Dry cleaners, fumigant workers, metal degreasers, printers, rubber wax makers
Polybrominated biphenyls (PBBs)	Fire-retardant makers
Polychlorinated biphenyls (PCBs)	Electric-capacitor makers and operators
Vinyl chloride	Polyvinyl-resin makers, rubber makers, organic-chemicals synthesizers
Estrogenic compounds	
Diethylstilbesterol	DES manufacturers, pharmaceutical workers
Other chemicals	
Carbon disulfide	Viscose rayon workers, degreasers, dry cleaners, carbon tetrachloride makers, paint workers, rocket fuel makers, rubber workers, textile makers, vacuum tube makers, grain fumigant workers
Ethylene oxide	Antifreeze-production workers, chemical sterilizer operators, hospital workers (instrument sterilization), fumigant workers, chemical workers, epoxy-resin workers, grain elevator workers
Ethylene thiourea	Rubber workers, fungicide workers
Infectious agents	
Rubella, herpes virus, syphilis, cytomegalovirus	Health-care workers, social workers, teachers, laundry workers, animal handlers
Physical hazards	
Noise	Factory workers, musicians, bar employees, foundry workers, airport workers
Heat	Foundry and oven workers, bakers, glassblowers, miners
Ionizing radiation	X-ray technicians, health-care workers, nuclear energy workers, pharmaceutical workers, industrial radiographers, dental assistants, foundry inspectors, workers involved with radium and radiation
Microwaves	Automotive workers, food products workers, furniture and wood workers, glass fiber workers, paper products workers, plastics workers, microwave application workers, textile workers, rubber products workers

Source: Adapted from a table prepared by Kathleen Rest, M.P.A.

What to Do about a Hazardous Job Situation

By completing the Work History form on page 257, you can assess the extent to which your job puts you at risk, if in fact it does. Have your partner complete the form, too. Include any exposures outside of work: doing housework (cleaning agents, solvents), working in the garden (pesticides), taking care of children (lifting, infections), or engaging in leisure activities (photography, crafts). Show your Work History form to your health-care provider, and consider with him or her the steps you need to take to avoid any potentially dangerous situations.

If you discover that your job poses a hazard to your pregnancy, it is up to you to change the situation. Belonging to a union or employee organization may put you in a better negotiating position than if you have to negotiate by yourself. A safe job is your right, but it's not always an easy right to ensure. Early action is important because a hazardous work situation can have disastrous consequences early in pregnancy. If a transfer to a safer job is the answer, ask your health-care provider for a letter justifying a transfer.

Your Legal Rights

The Occupational Safety and Health Administration (OSHA) was established in 1970 to ensure that workers have a safe workplace. The "General Duty Clause" of OSHA's legislative charter protects the worker's right to a safe and healthful workplace. "Healthful" is interpreted to include protection of reproductive health. If you feel that your workplace violates this federal law, you can file a complaint by contacting your state OSHA, or if there is not one, the federal OSHA. Your complaint can be completely confidential, and you are protected from punitive action for filing a complaint.

You cannot be fired because you may become or are pregnant, and you are protected from losing seniority when you return to work after delivery. An employer cannot refuse to hire or promote you or to give you benefits that other workers enjoy because you are pregnant. These rights are protected by the Pregnancy Discrimination Act (P.L. 95–555), a federal law passed by Congress in 1978 as an amendment to Title VII of the 1964 Civil Rights Act. This law is enforced by the Equal Employment Opportunity Commission.

RECOMMENDED RESOURCES

American College of Obstetricians and Gynecologists Guidelines on Pregnancy and Work. DHEW-NIOSH Research Report #210-76-0159. Publication #78–118, Sept. 1977. These guidelines were written for the practicing physician.

Clearinghouse for Occupational Safety and Health Information, NIOSH, 4676 Columbia Parkway, Cincinnati, Ohio 45226. (Tel.: 513-684-8328.) Write this agency for information about a specific hazard.

Equal Employment Opportunity Commission, 2401 E Street, N.W., Washington, D.C. This is the federal commission that enforces the Pregnancy Discrimination Act. The EEOC has many field offices.

9 to 5 VDT Hotline: 800-521-VDTS (in Ohio, 800-522-VDTS). Call for current information about risks to video display terminal workers. You can order up to five copies of 9 to 5's VDT Bill of Rights.

Occupational Safety and Health Administration, U.S. Department of Labor, 200 Constitution Ave., N.W., Washington, D.C. 20216.

11 About Miscarriage

Miscarriage is an event people usually avoid talking about. However, many pregnancies *do* end in miscarriage, often shattering joyous expectations, though it should be kept in mind that a miscarriage can be followed by a successful pregnancy. Since the first trimester is when the death of a fetus most often occurs, you should be acquainted early in your pregnancy with the physical and emotional aspects of miscarriage. If you and your partner do indeed have to face this fatal complication in your pregnancy, some advance knowledge of what is involved may somewhat lessen the trauma.

The Frequency of Miscarriage

How many pregnancies miscarry? Estimates range from 10 to 75 percent—but the higher estimates relate primarily to pregnancies at so early a stage of development that they often go unrecognized. It appears that a large number of fertilized ova fail to implant in the uterus and are expelled as part of a monthly period. Thus it is estimated that as many as 75 percent of pregnancies end in miscarriage, with the termination of the pregnancy usually not distinguishable from a regular period. Among women who have had enough time to learn they are pregnant (as a rule, about two weeks after missing a period), about 15 percent will miscarry. So, miscarriage is a real possibility in pregnancy.

Almost all miscarriages occur in the first trimester, within about ten weeks of conception. That is why many people decide not to spread the news about their pregnancy until the second trimester.

It probably is a good idea not to begin making specific plans for labor, delivery, and taking the new baby home until the first trimester is over.

Terminology

The stage of pregnancy at which a miscarriage occurs will determine how it will be officially recorded. You should know that neither the legal nor the medical profession uses the word "miscarriage" in its official nomenclature.

In legal terminology, any pregnancy that ends in the death of the fetus before 20 weeks from the last menstrual period, or before the baby weighs 500 grams (a little over a pound), is referred to as an "abortion." In medical terminology, a miscarriage is also called an abortion, or more precisely, a *spontaneous abortion*. (When a pregnancy is ended early by choice, the term used is *therapeutic abortion*.) Whenever there is significant bleeding during the first trimester, the medical profession speaks of a "threatened abortion," which means that a miscarriage may happen. If the membranes rupture or the cervix dilates, the abortion is referred to as "inevitable." From a legal standpoint, a miscarriage that occurs after the twentieth week is a "stillbirth," which must be documented with birth and death certificates.

Causes of Miscarriage

In almost every situation where a pregnancy ends in miscarriage, the developing fetus has died sometime before the miscarriage occurs. Frequently, the death occurs days or even weeks before the miscarriage. Thus miscarriage is the body's way of ridding itself of a pregnancy that has not developed normally. Microscopic studies have shown that often there is some obvious abnormality in the fetus or placenta. Between 50 and 60 percent of miscarriages have genetic (chromosomal) defects. Others occur clearly because of abnormalities of the placenta, infection, chronic disease in the mother, or exposure to harmful chemicals. A miscarriage can therefore be properly considered part of nature's way of helping assure that only healthy babies are born.

The Signs of Miscarriage

The first sign of miscarriage is usually bleeding from the vagina. Vaginal bleeding during pregnancy is not a sure sign of miscarriage; about 25 percent of pregnancies involve some spotting or heavier bleeding, and less than half of those do miscarry.

The other early sign of miscarriage is cramping in the lower abdomen. This often resembles a menstrual period, but it may be rhythmic like labor or feel like a low backache.

If both bleeding and pain are present, miscarriage is quite likely, but not inevitable. If clear or bloody fluid suddenly flows from the vagina, the bag of waters has probably broken and a miscarriage will almost certainly occur. When the miscarriage happens, a quantity of tissue is pushed from the uterus into the vagina. This tissue represents the remains of the membranes, placenta, and fetus. As it is pushed into the vagina, one usually feels a gush of blood, and within a few minutes the cramping subsides.

What to Do If Signs of Miscarriage Occur

If you develop the typical signs of miscarriage—bleeding and lower abdominal cramps—some physicians recommend that you limit your activities. Others, recognizing that miscarriage usually ends an abnormal pregnancy, do not recommend any treatment.

Since contractions and blood loss can be signs of potential miscarriage, you should stay in close communication with your health-care provider if they occur. Here are some guidelines for what to do:

- If mild bleeding or cramping occurs in the first trimester, call your health-care provider within a day and notify him or her of what has happened.
- If severe bleeding (like a period or heavier) occurs, call your health-care provider that day. He or she will probably want to see you in the office.
- If bleeding *and* cramping or lower abdominal pain occur, call your health-care provider and plan on being seen at his or her office or in the emergency room.
- If bleeding and cramping or lower abdominal pain are accompanied by a gush of water or passage of tissue, save any tissue that is passed. See your health-care provider within a few hours, bringing the tissue with you.
- If bleeding and cramping have been going on for some time and fever develops, see your health-care provider within a few hours.

The Medical Treatment of Miscarriage

Physicians and midwives take a "wait and see" approach when symptoms of miscarriage occur in early pregnancy. In nearly all instances of bleeding and cramping, they will wait for signs that the fetus has died or that miscarriage is inevitable before advising any treatment other than rest. This approach is used because many pregnant women who have apparent symptoms of miscarriage go on to deliver healthy, full-size babies.

Should you develop early signs of miscarriage, your health-care provider may do a pregnancy test, since pregnancy tests turn negative a week or so after the death of a fetus. If your pregnancy is more than two months old, your health-care provider may request an ultrasound. By about nine weeks, signs of fetal life (heartbeat and movement) can be noted on a sonogram. Lack of movement or a heartbeat when they should be apparent by ultrasound suggests that a miscarriage is likely to occur.

When a miscarriage does occur, it may be that the fetus and membranes are expelled but the placenta or a part of it remains inside. This is particularly common after the tenth week. When the placenta or other portions of the pregnancy stay in the uterus, continued bleeding and infection can result. For this reason, tissue that fails to come out during a miscarriage must sometimes be removed. The removal of the remaining tissue involves dilating the cervix and cleaning the uterus with an instrument called a curette. Thus, after miscarriage, many women undergo the procedure of dilation and curettage, which is typically referred to as "D and C."

Recurrent Miscarriage

Most miscarriages happen because of some abnormality of fetal development that occurred purely by chance. Between 70 and 90 percent of miscarriages are followed by a successful pregnancy. Recurrent miscarriage (two or more in a row) is also mostly due to chance, but sometimes a specific cause can be identified medically.

Because miscarriage is so often due to chance, it is generally wise to wait until three in a row have occurred before having a medical evaluation to look for a cause. If you do need to be evaluated for recurrent miscarriage, your physician will look for hormonal, nutritional, and other chronic medical problems, for incompatibilities of blood type between father and mother, for chronic infection in the mother, for unusual emotional stress, and for certain anatomic abnormalities of the uterus and cervix. Medical evaluation and treatment will result in a normal pregnancy in 70 to 85 percent of women who have had three consecutive miscarriages. Thus, even after several miscarriages, your chance of having a normal, healthy baby is quite good.

If you have a miscarriage, your physician may recommend that you wait a short time before getting pregnant again. Many physicians, however, recommend that a woman who has miscarried go ahead and try to get pregnant as soon as she feels ready.

Tubal Pregnancy

When a pregnancy develops in one of the fallopian tubes, instead of in the wall of the uterus, it eventually leads to death of the fetus, to bleeding inside the abdomen, and to the need for surgery. Although the exact events are somewhat different, the experience of having a tubal pregnancy is very similar to having a miscarriage.

Here's what typically happens: About 1 percent of the time, the fertilized ovum implants in one of the fallopian tubes. This may happen to any woman but is particularly common in women with an IUD or who have had previous infections of the tube. The pregnancy seems normal for several weeks, although sometimes there is mild spotting from the vagina or a vague discomfort on one side of the pelvis.

The wall of the tube is too thin to support a growing pregnancy, however, and eventually blood begins to leak into the abdomen. This causes pain low in the pelvis, often on one side or the other. The pain can be quite mild at first, or it can appear suddenly as severe cramps. This situation will only worsen until the pregnancy is removed; so, once the diagnosis is made, an operation is always needed—often on an emergency basis—to remove the pregnancy and tube.

Physically, you recover from the operation in about six weeks, but it often takes longer to mourn the loss of the pregnancy. In addition, having had a fallopian tube removed makes it somewhat harder to get pregnant in the future, and as many as 20 percent of women are unable to conceive after a tubal pregnancy. The surgery itself leaves you with one fallopian tube, however. If that tube is healthy, you have a good chance of getting pregnant again—this time in the uterus—and having the baby without problems.

Emotional Aspects of Miscarriage

Although miscarriage is a common event, it is not discussed much. After all, few women expect it to happen to them, and when it does, many don't talk about their experiences. While there are support groups for new parents and classes for expectant parents, little help or information is available to couples who experience miscarriage.

Being aware of how commonly miscarriages occur, and that you are by no means alone in this difficult experience, can be comforting. But couples are often unprepared for the emotional trauma that accompanies a miscarriage. In the event you miscarry, it is important for you to understand that the feelings you have are normal and are a necessary part of the healing process.

When miscarriage occurs, the first reaction of many women is shock and disbelief. When it begins you may not comprehend that it is really happening to you. You didn't expect it; you may have suppressed any thought of the possibility. It's natural to feel frightened about the experience: it can be very scary. Uncertainty makes it even more frightening. You'll wonder what went wrong, if it will happen again, if you'll be able to have children, or if there was something you did to cause it. We cannot emphasize too often that the great majority of miscarriages are not preventable and, in fact, happen because there was something wrong with the embryo.

The apparent onset of a miscarriage is naturally a time of great stress: bleeding or cramping are occurring and you do not yet know whether your pregnancy will actually fail. Some couples describe this period of time, which can last for days and even weeks, as being "in limbo." There are signs of imminent miscarriage, but you are told to wait. This can be agonizing. If you are "in limbo," you'll need all the support and comfort you can get, from your partner, close family, or friends. Do everything possible to make yourself comfortable.

When miscarriage occurs, it is quite normal to be afraid to look at the blood clots and tissue you pass. However, by seeing what actually has come out of your body, you can deal with your fears and begin to accept the fact that your pregnancy is over. What you imagine is likely to be much worse than the reality of the situation.

While coping with the shock and physical discomfort, you also have to contend with the medical system—a system that can seem impersonal and frightening to someone going through a miscarriage. A familiarity with terminology, the medical procedures, and symptoms can help you face the situation. Don't hesitate to ask questions when they come to mind. Having an informed and supportive partner is very valuable. Although in recent years the health-care community has increasingly emphasized the need to assist parents with the emotional aspects of birth, relatively little has been accomplished in making other medical events as personal. Dealing with the medical system can leave you frustrated. Perhaps the best way to try to cope with this frustration is to ask for emotional support and comfort from your partner or a friend.

A great source of support for many women is a friend, mother, sister, or other relative who has been through a miscarriage herself and can understand what you are going through. If you don't have such a person to talk to, sharing your feelings with someone you are close to—partner, mother, pastor, or friend—can be just as helpful. It's important to realize that your partner will have strong feelings about the situation, too, and that these are not necessarily going to be the same as yours. He will need to talk, to have support, and to grieve just as you do.

The need of both partners to mourn the loss of a pregnancy is often not considered. In fact, grieving over your loss is a natural and healthy reaction; give yourself time to experience it. The grieving process takes a while—sometimes months. When you feel sadness, instead of trying to push it aside, accept the appropriateness of the feeling. You have lost something very precious to you, and acceptance of the loss will allow you to go through the natural progression of feelings involved in the mourning process.

Telling People

If you told friends and relatives you were pregnant, you now have the task of telling them about the miscarriage. There will be people with whom you would prefer not to discuss the details; you needn't feel compelled to do so. If people offer unsolicited advice or theories about the cause of the miscarriage, you can tell them firmly that you understand they have your interest at heart but that you would rather not talk about it.

Your children are another matter. Young children will need a simple explanation, probably repeated over and over. Even though our natural reaction is to want to protect them from sadness, children will sense that something is wrong and will need reassurance from you. They should be told, in words you are comfortable with, that there was something wrong with the growing baby that made it impossible for you to stay pregnant, and that you don't understand it completely either. Seeing that there is sadness in life, but that we, as adults, cope with it and go on, is a strengthening experience for even the youngest child.

Remember: Miscarriages are far more common than most people realize, and the vast majority of women who suffer a miscarriage go on to become pregnant again, and to have healthy babies.

RECOMMENDED READING

Pizer, Hank, and Christine Palinski. *Coping with Miscarriage.* St. Louis: Mosby Books, 1983. An excellent, in-depth discussion of what happens during miscarriage and how to recover from it.

12 Emotions and Sexuality, 1

Pregnancy can be a shared experience involving more than just the physical circumstance of a woman carrying a fetus. You and your partner have a new bond—the prospect of a child—and that bond will naturally have an effect on your feelings, including your sense of sexuality. Each of you will view the events of pregnancy from a different angle. While an expectant mother undergoes physical changes that influence how she feels about herself and the world around her, the father-to-be is likely to experience emotional changes of his own that should be recognized and shared.

Throughout pregnancy and the postpartum period, it's important that both of you be aware of your own emotional needs and of ways to cope with the changes you will encounter. In a real sense, you are each "expecting"—and how you and your partner handle your expectations can make a difference in the quality of your pregnancy.

THE EXPECTANT MOTHER

As you become conscious of physical changes, keep in mind two important considerations: that emotional changes during this time are *normal* and are felt to some degree by all pregnant woman, and that you should *talk* about your feelings—with your partner, your doctor, your friends, or a counselor.

Many factors in your life can color your emotional outlook during pregnancy: the timing of the pregnancy, your relationship with your partner, whether this is your first pregnancy, as well as your

age, economic situation, and job status. But your emotional outlook is also tied to the physical changes you're going through; both
increased hormone production and physical discomfort can affect
your mood. Like most pregnant women, your emotions will probably be focused on specific concerns: self-image (it will certainly go
through some changes!), job and career, finances, your relationship with your partner (including your sex life), getting ready for
the baby, and thinking about the responsibility of becoming a
mother.

Pregnancy is a major transition in life, and having such concerns
is normal and healthy. It's one of the ways to prepare for change.

Body Image

As you experience the physical transformations of pregnancy, it's
natural for you to respond by having some new feelings about your
body and your self. It's true that many women feel more feminine,
more attractive, and sexier during their pregnancies than at any
other time. But many pregnant women also go through spells
when they feel less attractive. The feeling that you have lost control
of your body is common in the first trimester. When you are nauseated and tired, you may wonder where your energetic self has
gone. At those times, it's important to remind yourself (over and
over again if necessary!) that your pregnancy is temporary and that
your body will start to return to normal in just a few months.

Lifestyle Changes

When your pregnancy is confirmed, you'll no doubt wonder how it
will affect your career, your financial situation, and your relationship with your partner. These are practical concerns because having a baby will change your life drastically. It's sensible to start
thinking early in pregnancy about how you will adjust to new responsibilities and needs. Sometimes talking about plans, making
lists, reading books about starting a family, and getting yourself
emotionally ready for change will help to alleviate your concerns.
During the first trimester, give yourself time to consider your hopes
and intentions. You have many practical matters to think through,
but you needn't be overwhelmed: you still have seven or eight
months to work out many of the details.

Other Children

If you already have children, you've probably gotten lots of advice on when and how to announce your pregnancy to them. Of course, you're the best judge of that. In general, it's probably wise to inform them as early as possible. Even pre-verbal children will pick up on changes in your body and moods; verbal children may hear you talking about the pregnancy or hear the news from adults who assume they've been told. Like adults, children will exhibit a range of emotions: boredom, fascination, excitement, pride, worry about Mom. Allow your children to express their feelings; it's important for them to recognize and react to change.

Play is a good way for you to tune in to your children's feelings. Let their questions guide you in giving information. Often children will repeat questions several times. Keep your answers simple. There are many excellent books for children on pregnancy, birth, and feelings associated with having a new baby brother or sister.

Fantasies

Fantasies are particularly common during pregnancy and quite normal. You may find yourself dreaming about the future. Conversely, you may become obsessed with the past, perhaps with your childhood or with any unresolved losses or grief you might have. Your dreams, thoughts, and fantasies are all tools that help your psyche cope with and grow from pregnancy. Don't be afraid to examine them and, if you are comfortable enough, to talk about them. You may want to start a journal for recording your thoughts and fantasies.

Ambivalence about pregnancy is hard for many women (or couples) to admit or accept, but many women do have some negative feelings about pregnancy or the baby-to-be. Even in the case of the most deliberately planned pregnancy, it's natural to have an occasional second thought. The decision to have a child carries large responsibilities; of course you are concerned that you have, indeed, made the "right" decision.

You and Your Partner

A major concern for most couples is how a baby will affect their relationship. Communication, always important in a relationship, becomes even more crucial during your pregnancy. Little misunderstandings or events can easily get blown out of proportion. While you need to let your partner know how you're feeling, you should be aware that he probably needs more support now, too. Support for each other can come in several forms: verbal, sexual, physical, and emotional. Be sure to set aside time for yourselves. Go to your prenatal visits and childbirth education classes as a couple, if possible; that is a good way to help your partner feel more involved in the pregnancy.

Sexuality

Pregnancy may affect your sexual relationship with your partner. Before you and your partner were expectant parents, you were lovers. A loving, supportive, enjoyable sex life is an important part of a good relationship, and with openness and flexibility it can continue throughout pregnancy. During the first trimester, nausea and tiredness may make you less interested. On the other hand, not having to worry about birth control, along with joy and excitement over the pregnancy, can make sex better. The important thing, again, is to communicate your feelings and desires to your partner and to be sensitive to his feelings. Also, keep in mind that sex doesn't always have to include intercourse. Massage, for example, can be a wonderful way of communicating love to your partner.

In the past, some people have questioned whether orgasm could set off a miscarriage or early labor, since contractions of the uterus occur during orgasm. In fact, it is quite common for uterine contractions to continue on and off for several hours after orgasm. This is normal, and any association between orgasm and labor is probably coincidental.

If you have concerns about your sexual relationship that aren't covered in this book, be sure to bring them up with your health-care provider.

Your Support Systems

The support of your partner, family, and friends is important at any time, but their encouragement and concern are even more vital during pregnancy. Many pregnant women and expecting couples have found other pregnant women or couples to be sources of support. During the first trimester, you'll be aware that family and friends vary in their response to the news of your pregnancy. Some people may disappoint you; others may surprise you by their enthusiasm.

Sharing your feelings, experiences, and hopes with others who are going through a similar experience can be one of the best ways to relieve anxiety and get encouragement. It's fun to talk about the changes you are going through. You are fortunate, indeed, if you have friends who are pregnant or who have a new baby. By joining an "early bird" childbirth education class, you can enter into a valuable "support group." But if you don't have any sort of informal support network, you may wish to start a group of your own; two people are enough. The style is up to you. It can be informal, with no agenda, perhaps meeting for a potluck supper every week or two; or it can be a discussion group with topics to focus on each week. If you want names of other women who might be interested, ask your health-care provider or put up a notice at his or her office.

Once in a while, coping with changes related to a new pregnancy can get to be too much, especially if there have been complications or unusual stresses. If you are having trouble coping, take care of yourself just as you would for a purely physical problem: seek professional help. Among the symptoms that should lead you to seek professional help are listlessness (more than you'd expect during the first trimester), depression that doesn't go away after a few days, inability to relax, and withdrawal from family and friends. Start by consulting your health-care provider. He or she may want to recommend that you talk with someone else or may feel able to provide the extra support you need.

THE EXPECTANT FATHER

This section is particularly addressed to the father-to-be. As the lines between women's and men's roles have become less distinct, with women working outside the home, and men sharing child-care and household responsibilities, more attention is being paid to the part *you* play in starting and raising a family.

The extent to which you are an active participant in the pregnancy, birth, and infancy of your child is mostly determined by how you and your partner see your role, and by how active you yourself decide to be. The rigid thinking that once limited the father's responsibility to being provider and disciplinarian, but left him out of the emotional, day-to-day involvement with his family,

---

Changing Attitudes about the Father's Role

"Old"	"New"
Unemotional, in control, always on top of things	Able to express feelings, willing to share responsibility
Sole provider for family, carrying the burden of ensuring the welfare of wife and children	Options for sharing economic responsibility
Uninformed and uninvolved in decisions about childbirth, prenatal care, and early infant care	Well-informed, participates in decisions about birth and infant care
Leaves responsibility for child's upbringing to wife ("mothering is instinctive")	Both parents involved in care for infants and children
Must provide emotional support for wife, but may not ask for support	Seeks as well as provides support
Disciplinarian of children, rather than nurturer	Shares in the nurturing and disciplining of children

---

is fast disappearing. Expanding and defining your role in the family can strengthen your relationship with your partner and can give you opportunities to grow in ways you might never have imagined. The accompanying box details some of the attitudes about fatherhood that have changed in recent years.

During the first trimester, you and your partner are learning to accept the reality of the pregnancy and have the time to think about your changing roles. Now is when you can begin to accustom yourself to the thought of being more than a partner and lover. The transition to fatherhood can be enriching as well as confusing. If this is not your first child, you know something about what to expect. But each pregnancy stimulates new emotions, and you will want to be reassured as well as be reassuring in your relationship with your partner.

Emotional Swings

As an expectant father, you may experience emotional ups and downs and uncertainties, much as expectant mothers do. Aside from being the partner of someone who is going through an intense emotional and physical experience, you are going through an intense emotional experience of your own, one that may have physical implications. In some cultures, there is a syndrome called couvade (from the French *couver*, to brood or hatch), which manifests itself when a man experiences symptoms similar to his pregnant partner's. In our culture, couvade can take the form of emotional upheavals. When they occur, these feelings should be acknowledged, and discussing them with your partner can bring the two of you closer together. While your partner may need much emotional support, you may too, and it's important for your needs to be met.

Jealousy

Jealousy of pregnancy and of all the attention the pregnant woman gets is a common reaction—one that may crop up throughout pregnancy, and into the postpartum period. It's natural—don't deny the feeling if you have it. Sometimes just acknowledging that jealousy is there, and that it is a natural reaction, will help you cope with it.

Lifestyle and Finances

Your lifestyle may already have been affected by the pregnancy. Your partner may be feeling more tired and less willing to do the things the two of you have enjoyed as a couple. Understandably, you may feel concerned about finances now; and you may find your time and attention diverted to the coming baby more and more. If finances and changes in your daily routine weigh on your thoughts, discuss them with your partner. Keeping the lines of communication open is critical.

RECOMMENDED RESOURCES

Bittman, S., and S. R. Zalk. *Expectant Fathers*. New York: Ballantine Books, 1978. Written with sensitivity, this book emphasizes preparation for fatherhood and the choices expectant fathers can make to define their roles. There are many anecdotes from interviews with new and expectant fathers.

Fagerstrom, G., and G. Hansson. *Our New Baby: A Picture Story about Birth for Parents and Children*. Woodbury, N.J.: Barron's Educational Series, 1982. The story of a year in the life of one family during which a new baby is born. The range of emotions—including anger, joy, and jealousy—is discussed, and there are details about how the baby was conceived and born.

Nilsson, Lenart. *How Was I Born?* New York: Delacorte Press, 1975. Illustrated with Nilsson's photographs of fetal development, this book is for reading with young children.

PART III

The Middle Three Months

14–26 WEEKS

The baby moves. Some time during the last few weeks or very soon now you feel a sudden knock from inside you, or perhaps a flutter of movement as if butterflies were beating their wings. You wonder if it really can be the baby or if it is only your imagination. You have felt *life*. Another being is nestled deep in your body, shielded from harm, floating in an inner sea, swimming and turning, twisting and sometimes somersaulting.

—Sheila Kitzinger, *The Birth Diary*

For many women, the middle three months are the best part of the pregnancy; they tend to be a time of high energy and good feelings. The nausea and tiredness have faded, and the risk of miscarriage is reduced. Now you can begin to make specific plans for the infant soon to enter your life.

You will feel your baby move for the first time, and you'll devote a lot of your thoughts to wondering what your baby will be like.

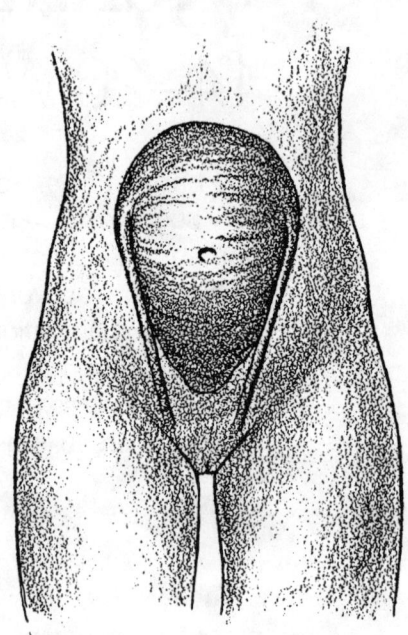

Fig. 31. Location of the round ligaments, which support the uterus and can cause lower abdominal pain in mid- or late pregnancy.

13 Common Body Changes in Pregnancy

As your pregnancy progresses, your body makes many adjustments to help the baby grow. Some of these happen without changing the way you feel or look. By the second trimester, however, you will probably have noticed many things about your body that are different. Some of the effects of pregnancy are quite bothersome, while others are no trouble at all. Such changes are normal and occur for explainable reasons, and you will find that many of the troublesome ones can be relieved. Some physical problems predictably increase and then lessen in intensity. During the middle three months, for example, you are likely to recoup your energies as the nausea and fatigue of early pregnancy wear off.

In this chapter, we discuss in alphabetical order the common body changes that can occur as a normal part of pregnancy. You will find both explanations and advice about these changes which may affect the way you feel and look.

Abdominal Pain

Lower abdominal pain is common in pregnancy, particularly in the second trimester. It has many causes, but the most common is round ligament pain. The round ligaments (see fig. 31) are actually muscles that hold the uterus upright. As the uterus grows, the round ligaments stretch more and more, becoming increasingly susceptible to strain. Pain along the ligament then results, often occurring or worsening when you move.

Rest is the best treatment, and pains usually subside quickly.

Good physical fitness through regular exercise helps prevent round ligament pain; it will provide added support for the uterus by keeping the abdominal wall muscles in good tone.

Backache

Several body changes during pregnancy may result in backache. As the uterus enlarges, it gradually alters your center of gravity and stretches the abdominal muscles. In addition, the ligaments and joints of your back and pelvis loosen during the last half of pregnancy. All these changes make it easy to pull or strain your back. If you do a lot of lifting—such as frequently picking up a young child—you are particularly likely to develop backache.

Having a sore back during pregnancy can be miserable, so take measures to prevent the problem from developing. Do your exercises regularly, wear comfortable shoes (flat or low-heeled shoes are best), and be sure you have a firm mattress. Instead of bending over, squat with your back straight. If your muscles ache at the end of the day, ask your partner to massage your back.

If you do develop backache, and it is bad enough to make you stop doing everyday activities, you should call your health-care provider. It is particularly important to get medical advice if back pain is accompanied by pain going down a leg or weakness in one or both legs.

Breast Changes

Early in pregnancy, breast tenderness, sensitivity of the nipples, and an increase in breast size occur as part of normal body adjustments. After the first few months, the breasts do not change significantly until early in the third trimester, when the milk glands begin to work. By the seventh month, the breasts produce small amounts of colostrum, a yellowish fluid your baby will drink during its first days of life. Darkening of the nipples also occurs during pregnancy.

These changes are normal. As your breasts increase in size, you should wear a larger, more supportive bra. If they begin leaking, place a cotton or gauze pad in each bra cup. Examine your breasts monthly for lumps, and report to your health-care provider any breast lump that does not go away in two weeks.

If you are planning to breastfeed your baby, you should prepare your breasts by toughening the sensitive skin of the nipple area.

This will prevent soreness and cracking of the nipples during the first ten days of breastfeeding. There are several ways to toughen the sensitive skin. Going without a bra part of each day allows the nipples to rub against your clothing. Rubbing the nipples with a washcloth or terrycloth towel for a minute or two during your bath is also helpful. Daily breast massage also works; your partner may be glad to help. Begin preparing your nipples about six weeks before your due date, and do something each day to make them less sensitive.

Breathing Difficulty

Shortness of breath is common in late pregnancy because the growing uterus takes up so much space that it limits the movement of the diaphragm. In addition, changes in the hormone (chemical) balance of your body during pregnancy cause a normal increase in breathing rate. These factors combine to make breathing feel more difficult. The feeling of being short of breath increases as pregnancy goes on. Some relief can occur in the ninth month, when the baby settles into the pelvis.

If you are having difficulty breathing, remember to stand and sit erect. When lying down, stay off your stomach, and try propping your head and shoulders on one or more pillows. To provide extra breathing space temporarily, raise your arms over your head. Another technique that helps is consciously breathing slowly and deeply. And, of course, avoid smoking.

Some shortness of breath is often unavoidable in late pregnancy. If you are unable to breathe comfortably even when propped up, have a rapid worsening of shortness of breath, or develop a persistant cough, you should definitely contact your health-care provider.

Circulation Changes

Changes in circulation during pregnancy are noticed mostly in the legs. As the uterus grows, it presses on the veins bringing blood back from the legs. This pressure slows the circulation in the legs, and standing or sitting for long periods of time aggravates the problem. The impaired circulation leads to leg fatigue. It commonly produces swelling of the ankles and feet, particularly after you have been standing for a long time. Also, the veins on the surface of the legs may bulge out, which is a condition called *varicose veins*. At night, poor circulation and lack of exercise can combine to cause painful leg cramps.

While these changes are common and are hard to prevent, there is a lot that can be done to make them less bothersome. Do daily exercises that stretch and move your leg muscles; they improve circulation, reduce fatigue, and prevent cramps. Avoid sitting or standing for long periods of time; walking will stimulate circulation. If your legs do swell or develop varicose veins, wear support stockings and avoid tight waistbands and elastic leg bands. You can reduce swelling during the day by elevating your legs for 30 to 45 minutes at midday.

Most circulatory problems during pregnancy will stay under control with exercise, support stockings, and leg elevation. There are, however, two situations that should lead you to promptly notify your health-care provider:

- **a varicose vein that becomes warm, hard, and painful** (suggesting phlebitis)
- **swelling that rapidly grows worse, particularly if the hands and face are involved** (suggesting preeclampsia)

Constipation

Constipation is quite common in pregnancy and probably has many causes. Iron or vitamin supplements, the need to drink additional water during pregnancy, pressure from the growing uterus on the intestines, and lack of exercise can all lead to constipation.

If you are having difficulty with constipation, these suggestions may help:

- Increase the fiber in your diet by eating raw vegetables, fruits, and whole grains. Bran (up to three tablespoons a day, mixed with cereal or any other moist food) and dried fruits (such as prunes or dates) are also helpful.
  - Drink at least two quarts (eight glasses) of fluid daily.
  - Be sure to exercise every day; walking is particularly helpful.
  - When you do feel the urge to have a bowel movement, don't put it off.

If the suggestions listed above do not work, and constipation remains bothersome, ask your health-care provider for advice.

Contractions

Tightening of the muscles of the uterus (Braxton Hicks or false labor contractions) occurs in all pregnancies after about 20 weeks.

These contractions generally last about one minute and come at irregular intervals. Some women are unaware of these contractions throughout pregnancy, but for others they can be severe enough to be quite painful.

If you notice these contractions, you should continue going about your everyday activities. What is happening is quite normal: the uterus is practicing for labor. If the contractions are particularly bothersome, you need to relax or lie down for relief.

While contractions are normal throughout the last half of pregnancy, you must be able to tell the difference between Braxton Hicks contractions and labor. Going into labor before the ninth month is a serious situation and should be reported right away to your health-care provider. You should, therefore, become familiar with the signs of early labor, which are discussed in detail on page 148.

Hair Changes

Your hair can change in unpredictable ways during pregnancy. Many women notice no changes at all. Often, however, hair becomes more difficult to set and will not keep a permanent. Some women find that their hair and eyebrows thin out. These changes are temporary, and after pregnancy hair returns to normal.

If your hair thins or will not keep a set well, readjust your hairstyle to best fit the change. We recommend that you avoid hair dyes in the first trimester because it is uncertain whether all colorings are safe during that period.

Headaches

Headaches are quite common in pregnancy. Some women suffer from daily headaches, while others have only one or two—or none at all. Some of these headaches are clearly "sinus" type, caused by increased blood flow and swelling of the nose and sinus region, which can also lead to nasal stuffiness. Other headaches occur for less clear reasons, perhaps fatigue, tension, eyestrain, or hormonal changes.

If you are having trouble with headaches, acetaminophen (Tylenol, Datril) is safe to take, even early in pregnancy. Some physicians recommend that aspirin not be used during the first trimester; most advise women in the third trimester that they not take aspirin because it slows blood clotting. Sinus headaches often respond to a warm shower or to a warm washcloth placed over the nose and eyes. Tension and tiredness will worsen headaches; so, rest and relaxation are often helpful.

If you have frequent headaches or feel you need to take more than four aspirin or acetaminophen pills a day, you should talk this over with your health-care provider. Headaches accompanied by dizziness, blurred vision, or spots before your eyes may be a sign of preeclampsia, particularly in the last half of pregnancy, and they should be reported.

Heartburn

Heartburn is an uncomfortable fullness, ache, or burning feeling in the lower chest, behind the breastbone. It occurs when stomach acid leaks into the lower esophagus. In pregnancy, hormonal changes relax the muscle at the top of the stomach that blocks acid flow into the esophagus. In addition, growth of the uterus causes pressure on the stomach, aggravating heartburn. In susceptible people, lying down after a meal is particularly likely to cause heartburn.

If you have trouble with heartburn, don't lie down when your stomach is full. Eat five or six small meals a day, rather than a few large ones, and avoid spicy foods. If heartburn persists at night, prop yourself up with pillows or elevate the head of your bed on wooden blocks. Antacid medications are considered safe after the first trimester and can be most helpful. If these measures do not provide relief, talk with your health-care provider.

Hemorrhoids

Hemorrhoids are normal veins in the area of the rectum. They often become enlarged in late pregnancy because there's more blood flowing through them, and the enlarged uterus makes it more difficult for blood to circulate in the rectal area. Sometimes, hemorrhoids become worse right after delivery. A swollen hemorrhoid can ache, become quite painful, and bleed, but most hemorrhoids are only mildly irritating.

Some simple things may help prevent hemorrhoids. Constipation and straining for bowel movements should be avoided. In addition, keeping good muscle tone in the rectal area by doing Kegel exercises may be helpful.

When hemorrhoids are tender, use wet baby wipes instead of toilet paper. Sitting in a hot bath for 20 minutes, and then applying witch hazel to the affected area, will often relieve swollen, sore hemorrhoids. If a hemorrhoid becomes hard and very tender, or bleeds, you should contact your health-care provider.

Nasal Stuffiness

Increased circulation in the nasal area sometimes produces a constant stuffiness during pregnancy. This feeling is often described as having a "constant cold" and is due to normal hormonal changes. Women with allergies or sinus problems before being pregnant can have particular difficulty with stuffiness.

Sometimes an increase in humidity helps; try using a vaporizer. Medications should generally be avoided, since stuffiness is likely to be present throughout much of pregnancy. If you are miserable, however, talk with your health-care provider. There are a number of medications that can be safely used in pregnancy.

Nausea and Vomiting (Morning Sickness)

In general, the severity of nausea and vomiting peaks by the third month of pregnancy; thereafter, your stomach should feel more settled. During the first trimester, "morning sickness" can occur throughout the day, particularly when the stomach is empty.

Here are some tips for surviving the nausea of early pregnancy:

• Having something in your stomach often relieves morning sickness. If nausea is a problem when you awaken, keep some crackers at your bedside and eat them before you get up. Eat small but frequent amounts of food during the day.

• Avoid sudden movements when you are nauseated.

• Make sure you are drinking plenty of fluids. Popsicles, jello, and juices often serve the purpose well.

• Cooking meals can be miserable when you are nauseated, and grease and other odors are particularly bothersome. Opening windows and using the fan while you're cooking can help.

If you find that you are nauseated much of the day, in spite of taking the measures we've listed above, talk to your health-care provider about medication. If you can't keep liquids down, contact your health-care provider right away.

Nose and Gum Bleeding

Circulation to the nose and gums increases during pregnancy. As a result, nosebleeds and tender, bleeding gums are common.

If you develop a nosebleed, pinch the nose tightly for five minutes. Dryness in the nose can lead to nosebleeds; one effective remedy is to gently swab the inside of your nose with a Q-tip coated with petroleum jelly.

For bleeding gums, use a soft toothbrush and mild toothpaste. Floss your teeth daily; at first, there will be some bleeding, but the gums will soon grow healthy and strong. Rinsing your mouth with warm salt water can relieve swollen gums.

A nosebleed that you are unable to stop will need medical attention. Severe gum swelling and tenderness, or tooth pain, should be reported to your dentist. Pregnancy is not a reason to avoid dental work, but do tell your dentist that you are pregnant.

Skin Changes

A number of skin changes can be observed in pregnancy. Darkening of some areas is common, due to higher levels of a certain hormone that increases skin pigment. Many women notice darkening of the nipples and of a line that goes up the middle of their stomachs from the pubic area to the belly button. The skin tends to be oilier, which sometimes worsens or brings on acne. Unexplained rashes can occur. Moles may darken, and small red blotches may crop up on the arms, chest, and face. Also, some women develop a reddish or brown area over the bridge of the nose and below the eyes, which is sometimes referred to as the "mask of pregnancy." As fat is deposited on the hips and the abdomen grows, stretch marks may appear. Itching is also sometimes a problem during pregnancy.

All these skin changes are harmless. With the exception of stretch marks, most will go away after pregnancy, although they may take six to twelve months to do so.

There is no proven way to prevent stretch marks. Some people recommend massaging the hips and abdomen daily with cocoa butter, vitamin E, or some other lotion. It may not work, but at least it feels good. Because skin tends to be oilier during pregnancy, you may need to bathe and shampoo more often.

If a mole changes color or rapidly increases in size, point it out to your health-care provider.

Tiredness and Faintness

The Hollywood stereotype of the swooning pregnant lady has its basis in fact. Loss of energy, due to hormonal changes, is very common in early pregnancy. A tendency to become dizzy or faint can result from this tiredness and from a lowering of blood pressure that may occur in pregnancy. These feelings often fade by the second trimester. In the last few months, however, energy again diminishes.

The best way to combat tiredness is to get more rest. If you can, take a nap or lie down at least once during the day. If you work full-time, try to find a place to relax during the lunch hour. When you get home from work, allow yourself to rest instead of immediately starting dinner. Regular exercise helps, too; it will keep your stamina up and make you feel healthier.

If you feel persistently worn out, ask your health-care provider to check you for anemia.

Urination Problems

Frequent trips to the bathroom are definitely part of being pregnant. The cause is pressure of the uterus on the bladder, which limits the ability of the bladder to fill with urine. This pressure is particularly noticeable in the first trimester, when the uterus grows entirely within your pelvis, and in the third trimester, when the uterus is quite large. The result is a frequent need to urinate.

Because this is a normal body change, you should accommodate it by visiting the restroom as often as you feel you need to. Do *not* limit your fluid intake, since drinking plenty of fluids is important in pregnancy. If you notice burning or pain when you urinate, you may have a bladder infection and should contact your health-care provider.

Many pregnant women have difficulty holding their urine when they cough, sneeze, or laugh. This is particularly common late in pregnancy, and among women who have been pregnant before. The cause is poor muscle tone in the area supporting the bladder.

Often, this problem can be prevented or alleviated by doing Kegel exercises frequently. Many women who have this problem carry a change of underwear or wear a small pad when they go out. It nearly always stops after your baby is born.

Vaginal Discharge

An increased amount of vaginal discharge is normal in pregnancy. This discharge is due to hormonal changes and increased blood flow to the vagina. The discharge itself is whitish and may be thick or thin; it is not symptomatic of a problem.

If the discharge is leaking out during the day, carry a change of underwear or use a small pad. Bathe daily and carefully, but avoid douching. To prevent yeast infections (monilia), which are common in pregnancy, keep the groin area cool and dry by wearing skirts and cotton underwear.

You may develop a vaginal infection while you are pregnant. Itching, burning, or swelling of your labia may be signs of infection and should be reported to your health-care provider. An unpleasant vaginal odor should also be reported. If you suddenly develop a large amount of watery discharge, especially if you're in the third trimester, your bag of waters may be leaking; call your health-care provider.

14 Travel during Pregnancy

In general, if your health is good, there is no reason not to travel during pregnancy. The developing fetus is well protected, and you will not damage the baby or cause miscarriage by traveling on a bumpy or prolonged trip. In the first trimester, precautions need to be taken to avoid fatigue and nausea. The second trimester, however, is an excellent time to travel: complications are relatively few, and most women have a lot of energy during these months. We recommend that couples consider getting away for a vacation during the middle three months because they may not have many chances to relax together once the baby is born.

Comfort and Precautions

The main hazards of traveling during pregnancy are fatigue and backache. Keep up a regular exercise program, don't overstrain when carrying luggage, and allow for a period of rest during the day. In the last half of pregnancy, the large size of the uterus can restrict blood flow back from the legs, which can lead to swelling and to the possibility of blood clots forming. You can avoid circulatory problems while traveling by not sitting for too long a spell. In a plane, get up periodically and walk for a minute or two. If you are driving, stop every hour and stretch your legs.

As you get closer to your anticipated due date, make your trips away from home shorter. We recommend that in the last two months of pregnancy you limit travel to places within a two- or (at most) three-hour drive from home.

When traveling by car, remember to wear your seat belt and shoulder strap. You may have heard that wearing a seat belt is unsafe in pregnancy because it can injure the uterus during a collision. While this has happened a few times, you are far more likely to injure yourself and the fetus by *not* wearing a seat belt. Wear the shoulder harness as well; it will protect you better and will take much of the pressure off your abdomen if you are in an accident.

If you plan to travel by plane, here are some tips that may make your trip more comfortable:

- To avoid standing in line, buy your tickets and have your seat selection made in advance.
- Choose a seat in the nonsmoking section and, if possible, near a restroom.
- Every hour, get up and walk, to stretch your legs and stimulate circulation. You can also do stretching exercises in your seat.
- If you have nausea or don't like airplane meals, bring your own food in a traveling bag. Most airlines will allow you to order a vegetarian meal or a fresh-fruit plate when you make your reservation.
- Avoid long flights during the third trimester.
- If you do happen to develop contractions, or your water breaks while flying, don't panic. Remember that the average labor takes a lot longer than most flights. Tell one of the attendants about your situation, and then do your best to stay calm.

Immunizations

If you are planning a trip abroad and will be pregnant or trying to get pregnant, you should be aware of the risks of immunizations and other preventive measures.

The two immunizations that are believed to be the safest for pregnant women are tetanus shots and gamma globulin (used to prevent hepatitis). Both are without any known risk during pregnancy.

Yellow fever vaccine and the oral polio virus immunization seem to be relatively safe. Both are living viruses, however, and may pose some risk, particularly in the first trimester. For this reason, you should avoid traveling to places where you need these immunizations. But if you must travel to a high-risk area, it is better to get the immunization than to chance getting the disease.

Typoid and cholera vaccines are of unknown safety when given during pregnancy. Neither is a particularly effective vaccine anyway, and both have bothersome side effects. You should not have these immunizations during pregnancy. A few countries require some cholera immunization (usually just one shot) before entry. If you must travel to such an area, have your physician write a letter on letterhead stationery stating that, for medical reasons, you should not receive the immunization. That usually gets you through.

Malaria prevention is a particularly troublesome topic. Chloroquine is the drug usually taken to prevent malaria, and it is considered safe for the fetus in the dosages used. However, many areas of the world now have chloroquine-resistant strains of malaria. The alternative drug, a combination of pyrimethamine and sulfadoxine, is *not* safe during pregnancy. Therefore, women who are pregnant or likely to become so should avoid traveling to areas with chloroquine-resistant malaria.

Be Prepared for a Medical Problem

Take into account that a medical problem may occur while you're away from home. To prepare for this possibility, you should discuss your travel plans with your health-care provider. Ask for a copy of your prenatal record, or have your health-care provider complete the Prenatal Summary for Travelers on page 258. If your pregnancy has medical complications, ask your physician about the safety of any anticipated trip.

15 Emotions and Sexuality, 2

For the expectant mother, the middle three months of pregnancy are often a high point psychologically and physically. For the expectant father, the reality of the pregnancy is undeniable, yet perhaps still hard to grasp. For both, the second trimester involves a new intensity of emotion and, in many cases, of sexuality as well.

THE EXPECTANT MOTHER

You're now used to the idea that you will have a child; you're probably over the worst of your nausea and exhaustion; and you're finally *looking* pregnant.

Quickening

Sometime during these months (between about the fourteenth and twenty-second weeks) you will feel the baby move for the first time. This awareness of the baby's movement is called quickening. It makes the baby seem more real inside of you, and strong emotions may be associated with it. Many women feel tremendously excited by these first tiny flickerings. But the sudden sign of new life can be unsettling. Feeling this living thing inside of you, moving on its own, can make you reflect about the responsibilities of parenthood. Your partner may not be able to feel movement right away; but soon he, too, will share in this exciting event, and it may make him feel more involved in your pregnancy. Whatever your first reactions are, you'll be more aware than ever of your pregnancy and of its implications. And most likely you'll enjoy the sensation of feeling your baby move.

Sexuality

Studies have shown the middle months to be a sexual high, even surpassing the prepregnant state. Why? Perhaps because you feel better and have a lot of energy. You don't have to worry about birth control, and your abdomen still isn't too large to interfere. Many couples find that during this stage of the pregnancy their sexual relationship is better than ever. By all means, take advantage of the time you have together and explore your heightened awareness of each other.

For most women, growth of the uterus and tenderness of the breasts eventually make the traditional lovemaking position (with the man on top) uncomfortable. By experimenting with different positions—such as propping yourself up with pillows, lying side-by-side, or with the man entering from behind—a couple can enjoy intercourse (if desired) right up to the time of labor.

Body Image

Instead of looking just plump, you're beginning to look "definitely pregnant," and you are probably wearing maternity clothes by now. You may feel proud of your new image, but you may also feel self-conscious. There's no more hiding the fact of your pregnancy, even from strangers on the street. Friends and family will comment on your more obviously pregnant self, too. You may enjoy their attention, but you may also find yourself irritated by the continuing flow of comments.

Amniocentesis

If you are to undergo amniocentesis, there will be emotional as well as physical factors to consider. Couples usually understand what physically happens during the procedure (it will be explained carefully to you) but are unprepared emotionally for what the procedure entails. You should know that you will probably have to wait two to three weeks to get a final report from the laboratory. When there's so much emotional involvement in the results of a medical test, any lapse of time can seem excrutiatingly long. Difficult, too, is the fact that you'll become more and more attached to the growing fetus as you wait. Be aware that the wait will be a stressful time for both you and your partner. Ask for as much support as you require to take care of your emotional and psychological needs. Don't be afraid to discuss your fears and fantasies.

Worries and Concerns

Your concerns during the middle months are likely to focus on several areas. You may be thinking about what the baby will be like, if he or she will be healthy, what labor and delivery will be like, and whether you'll be able to cope with being a mother. It's normal to be concerned about these things; talk about your feelings with people you're close to. These normal concerns may manifest themselves in fantasies or dreams, and this, too, is normal.

If you're not involved in a group with other pregnant women or couples, now is a good time to find one. You can start one yourself if there isn't one available. You'll find plenty to talk about.

Relatives

Your parents and in-laws may start to question you about your plans for the baby's birth, names, whether you'll breastfeed, and so on. If you are undecided or just don't want to talk about your plans, you may not appreciate their curiosity. Without causing unnecessary hard feelings, you can tell them that, while you are thinking about these things, you are not quite ready to discuss your intentions. Remember that your pregnancy is a time of transition for your parents and in-laws, too, particularly if it is your first. Their child is about to become a parent, and they will be grandparents. All of this change can be a stress on your relationship with them. Communication is now crucial, even if stressful.

Personal and Couple Self-Care

As your pregnancy continues, keep in mind the two most important things you can do to ensure your emotional well-being and that of your partner:

- Recognize that feelings are normal and healthy and that your feelings, however strong, are shared to some extent by all pregnant women.
- Talk about your feelings with your partner, with your friends, and with whomever you feel comfortable.

THE EXPECTANT FATHER

During the second trimester, you will see your partner's abdomen enlarge to the point that she really looks pregnant. And this is the trimester when *you* feel the baby move for the first time. The experience of feeling your baby move can invoke deep feelings, ranging from panic ("My God, I *am* going to be a father!") to exhiliration, to an almost spiritual awe. Whatever your reaction, be prepared for an intense moment!

As your partner's abdomen grows and becomes more noticeably pregnant, you can expect to have varying feelings about her changing body. You may at times find her voluptuous and sexy; or on occasion simply fat. Some men are fascinated with the physical process from beginning to end, others less so. All of these reactions are normal. What is most important is that you be aware of your own feelings and realize that they will probably fluctuate.

This is also the time in pregnancy when women are notoriously sexual. There's some doubt as to how common this increased sexual desire is, but some women report having more intense sexual feelings during the second trimester than at any other time in their lives. For some men, it can be difficult to accept their partner's heightened sexuality: pregnancy and sex may not seem to belong together. If you feel uncomfortable, do talk to your partner about it. Try not to make her feel rejected, but express your concerns. A passionate woman can be very demanding, and at a time when you may have heightened sensitivities of your own, this can be especially hard to deal with.

You should also be aware that your partner may feel increasingly vulnerable. She may become anxious for your safety, have dreams about your being hurt or in danger, and generally "mother" you more than you would like. This is understandable—she is realizing how dependent on you she is right now.

If you have not been going with your partner to her regular prenatal checkups, you should consider starting to do so now. By attending these sessions, you will be more informed, you will feel more a part of the process of the pregnancy, and you can seek advice about any issues that concern you.

Soon it will be time for you and your partner to discuss childbirth education classes, and you will want to think about what your role will be during the labor and delivery. Whether or not you attend classes with your partner, you have the right to be present at the birth of your child. You don't have to make decisions now, but it's a good time to start talking about the final stages of pregnancy and the part you will play in them.

16 A Timeline of Fetal Growth

As you approach the last three months of pregnancy, the new being within you will often remind you of its presence. But you may not know how to visualize the stages of your baby's development. The growth from embryo to a fully matured infant is marked by distinctive transformations that occur in a predictable sequence. You have to picture first a tiny ball made up of cells and then imagine how the head, the hands, the feet, and other features begin to take on a recognizable shape. While you await the decisive moments of labor and delivery, time may seem to pass all too slowly; but the steady progression toward infancy—toward life that can breathe and move about outside of your safe, warm womb—is in fact remarkably fast. From the time you conceive, about 240 days go by, and suddenly you no longer need to imagine what your baby will look like.

The Developing Embryo at Four Weeks after the Last Menstrual Period

The chronology of a developing baby begins two weeks before fertilization and continues for approximately forty weeks, when the baby is born. For two weeks after the beginning of the last menstrual period, an ovum matures within the ovary. Approximately fourteen days after the last menstrual period, that ovum bursts free from the ovary, begins moving down the fallopian tube, and then is fertilized. Within a week of fertilization, the embryo develops into a microscopic ball of cells called a blastocyst (fig. 32). Initially all alike, the cells soon begin to differentiate into membranes, placenta, and the embryo itself. At the same time, the blastocyst attaches itself to the lining of the uterus.

The Developing Embryo at Seven Weeks

During weeks five through ten, most of the major organ systems of the body develop. By seven weeks, the embryo has begun to change from a straight oblong series of bumps to a folded over, vaguely humanoid shape (fig. 33). The heart has begun to beat, and blood cells have formed in the yolk sac, which protrudes from the developing abdomen of the embryo and soon will disappear. At seven weeks, the embryo is less than one-quarter inch long.

Fetal Growth between Nine and Twelve Weeks

By week twelve, all major organs have formed, and the embryo is about three inches long. Hands and feet are developing from tiny buds into stubby, but well-formed limbs (figs. 34 and 35). The embryo itself is beginning to look more like a person, with a huge head and tiny body.

The Head at Thirteen Weeks

At thirteen weeks, the embryo's head is large, round, and bald (fig. 36). Eyes are present, but the eyelids have not formed or opened. The ears are smooth bumps on the side of the head, and few facial features are present. There are no eyebrows or eyelashes.

The Fetus at Nineteen Weeks

By nineteen weeks, the body of the fetus has enlarged relative to the head (fig. 37). The fetus itself is about eight inches long. It is surrounded by amniotic fluid, the watery substance that protects it from injury and permits it to move. The arms and legs, which were originally quite stubby, have become almost normally proportioned. The ears are formed more distinctly, and there is a small amount of hair on the head. A cheesy material called vernix covers the delicate skin to protect it from becoming chapped.

The Fetus at Twenty-five Weeks

The fetus is now about ten inches long and weighs one-and-a-half pounds. Its skin is wrinkled and its body rather lean (fig. 38). Later on, fat will develop below the skin, giving the newborn its rounded appearance. In contrast, an infant born prematurely is skinny, with wrinkled skin. By the twenty-fifth week, the inner ear has completely developed, and the fetus will react to loud noises.

The Fetus at Thirty-five Weeks

By thirty-five weeks, the fetus is approaching its appearance at birth (fig. 39). It is approximately eighteen inches long and weighs between five and six pounds. The fingernails and toenails are still relatively short, and the ears are not as stiff as they will be at forty weeks. The eyelids, which have been sealed closed, can now open. By this time, many fetuses have settled into the head-down position that is ideal for birth.

Posture of a Mature Infant before Birth

At birth, the average newborn is around twenty inches long and weighs about seven-and-a-half pounds. Muscle tone is good, with arms and legs actively flexing. When still cramped in the uterus, however, the infant's arms and legs are folded so that they occupy the least possible space (fig. 40). Movements just before birth are limited to jerks and kicks of the folded arms and legs. Beneath the skin is a generous layer of fat, which provides insulation against the cold and gives the newborn its soft look.

TIMELINE OF GROWTH DURING PREGNANCY

WEEK	MOTHER BODY CHANGES OBSERVATIONS	BABY DEVELOPMENT ACTIVITIES	
1	● Last menstrual period.		
2	● Ovum grows within ovary. ● Ovulation occurs.	● Fertilization occurs in the fallopian tube.	
3	● The lining of the uterus becomes spongy as it prepares for implantation.	● The fertilized ovum has become a microscopic ball of cells called a blastocyst, which is ready to subdivide into a placenta, membranes, and an embryo. The blastocyst arrives in the uterus by the fourth day after fertilization.	
4	● Starting about the fourth week, symptoms of early pregnancy are noted—nausea, breast tenderness, tiredness. ● Mild bleeding from the vagina can accompany implantation.	● Implantation of the blastocyst into the wall of the uterus occurs. ● The placenta is beginning to develop.	
5	● First missed menstrual period. ● Serum pregnancy test becomes positive.	● Earliest beginnings of the embryo itself as a flat disk, which will fold, bend, grow, and develop into the baby. ● During the fifth and sixth weeks, the blood and vascular systems develop. ● The heart begins to beat.	
6	● Urine pregnancy test becomes positive.	● Early development of major organ systems, including brain, lungs, and liver, can be noted. ● The embryo is 4-5 millimeters long and weighs less than one-thirtieth of an ounce.	
7	● The uterus is the size of a large hen's egg. ● Frequent need to urinate is common due to pressure of the growing uterus on the bladder.	● The arms and legs are present as short buds on the embryo. ● The nose begins to form.	
8		● Fingers and toes are present.	
9		● Formation of the skeleton is complete. Calcium begins to be deposited by the end of the ninth week in the bones of the upper arm and continues to be deposited throughout pregnancy and childhood.	
10	● The uterus has grown to the size of an orange.	● Sometime during the tenth through twelfth weeks, the fetal heartbeat can be heard for the first time with an ultrasonic stethoscope (doptone).	

APPEARANCE OF GROWING FETUS

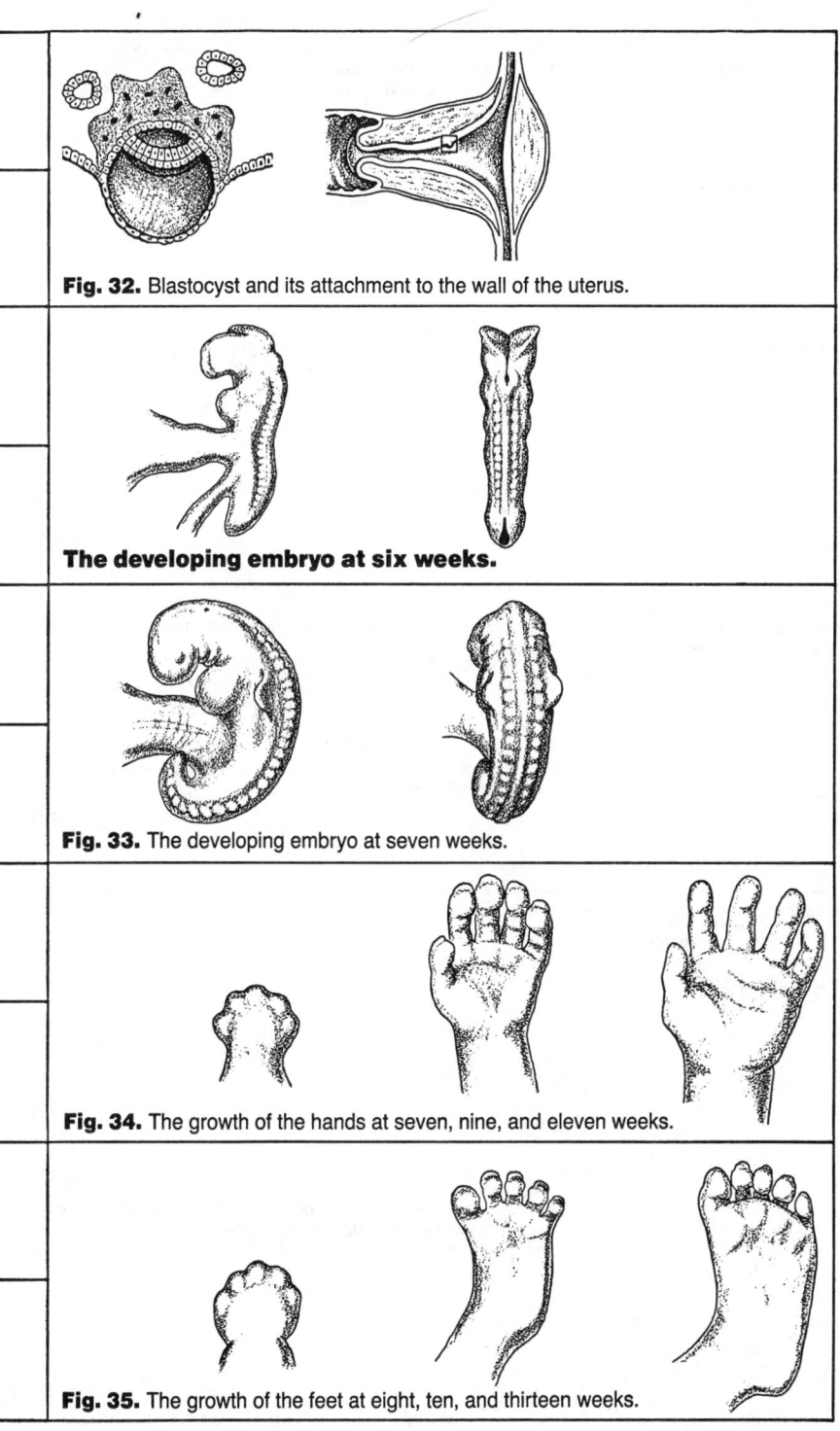

Fig. 32. Blastocyst and its attachment to the wall of the uterus.

The developing embryo at six weeks.

Fig. 33. The developing embryo at seven weeks.

Fig. 34. The growth of the hands at seven, nine, and eleven weeks.

Fig. 35. The growth of the feet at eight, ten, and thirteen weeks.

WEEK	MOTHER BODY CHANGES OBSERVATIONS	BABY DEVELOPMENT ACTIVITIES	
11	● The uterus can be felt for the first time above the pubic bone.	● During the eleventh and twelfth weeks, movements begin to occur, including kicking of legs, swallowing of amniotic fluid, and pursing of lips.	
12		● The fetus is about 3 inches long and weighs half an ounce.	
13	● The uterus is the size of a grapefruit.	● Formation of all major body parts is complete. Further development involves growth and refinement of all body structures.	
14	● Second trimester begins.	● During the fourteenth through sixteenth weeks, hair begins to develop on the head.	
15	● Women who have been pregnant before often note first fetal movements.	● The fetus is about 4-1/2 inches long and weighs about 2-1/2 ounces.	
16		● Genitals have developed to the extent that boys and girls can usually be told apart.	
17	● Colostrum production has begun. ● During the next two weeks, women who have not been pregnant before usually become aware of fetal movements.		
18			
19		● The arms and legs, which were initially quite short and stubby, have become normally proportioned. A cheesy material called vernix covers the delicate skin to protect it from abrasion and chapping while in the amniotic fluid.	
20	● The uterus reaches up to the level of the umbilicus.	● The fetal heartbeat can be heard with a fetoscope. ● The fetus is about 9 inches long and weighs about 8 ounces.	

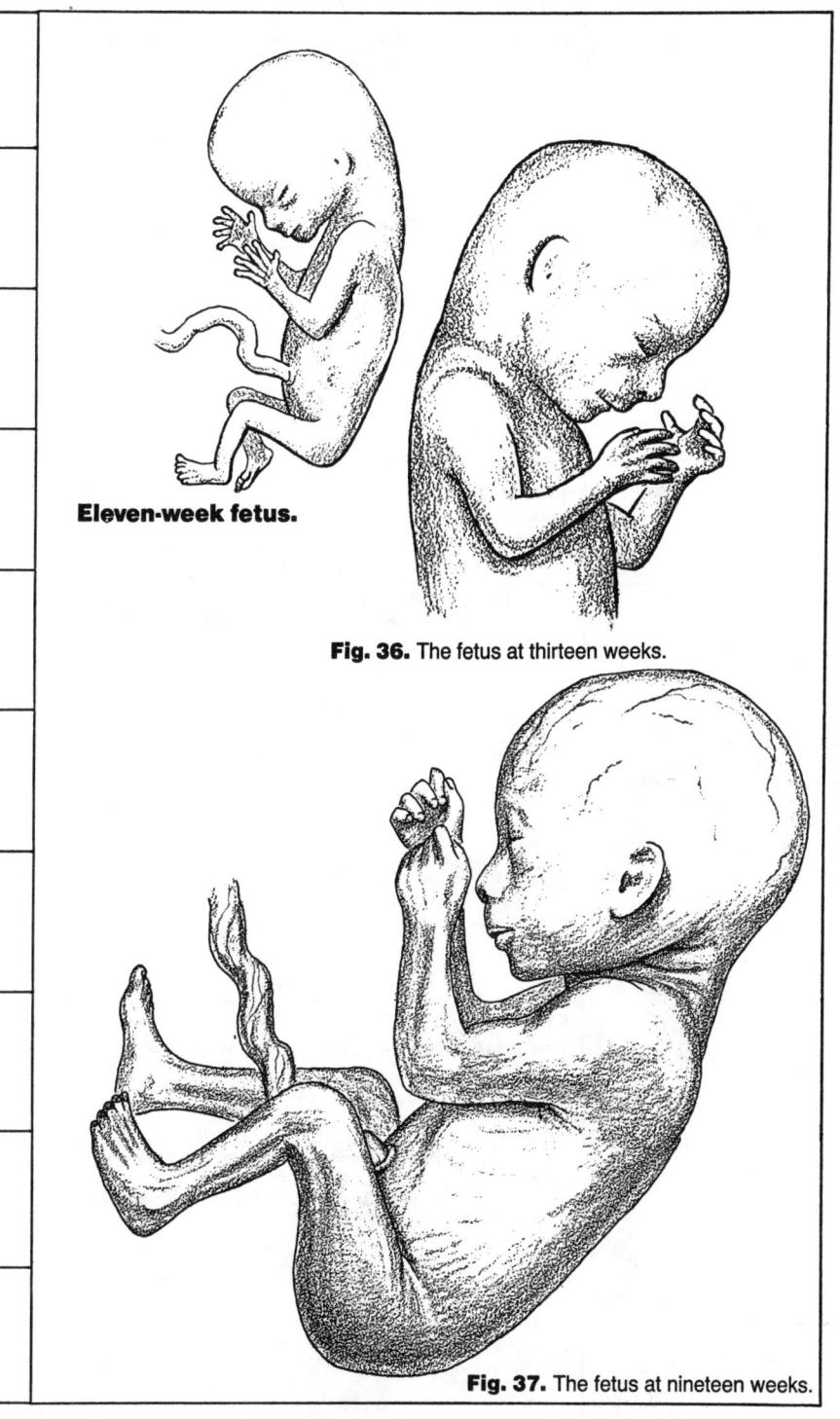

Eleven-week fetus.

Fig. 36. The fetus at thirteen weeks.

Fig. 37. The fetus at nineteen weeks.

WEEK	MOTHER BODY CHANGES OBSERVATIONS	BABY DEVELOPMENT ACTIVITIES
21	• Uterine (Braxton Hicks) contractions are often first felt about this time. • Pregnancy is half over!	• During the twenty-first through twenty-third weeks, considerable growth and weight gain occur.
22	• Blood pressure, which tends to be lower during much of pregnancy than at other times, reaches its lowest point. From now on, it will gradually rise until delivery.	• By this time, the inner ear is completely developed. The fetus is surrounded by constant loud, rhythmic sounds of blood flow. Occasionally, loud music, a door slamming, or other sounds from outside will reach the fetus and cause a noticeable reaction.
23		
24		• Eyebrows and eyelashes begin to become noticeable. • The fetus is about 12 inches long and weighs about 1-1/2 pounds.
25		• The skin is red and wrinkled, with little fat beneath it. (Later more fat will form, which makes newborns look pink.)
26	• Fetal movements and parts of the developing baby can be clearly felt within the abdomen. Often the doctor or midwife can identify where the head, back, and extremities are positioned.	
27	• Third trimester begins.	• Some fetuses can be observed sucking their thumb in the uterus by the seventh month.
28		• Beginnings of alertness can be noted. • The fetus is about 14 inches long and weighs about 2-1/4 pounds.
29		• Development has progressed enough so that nearly half of fetuses can, if born this early, survive with intensive care. Mortality rates decrease with each additional week of intrauterine growth and development.
30	• The uterus reaches about halfway between the umbilicus and the rib cage.	

APPEARANCE OF GROWING FETUS

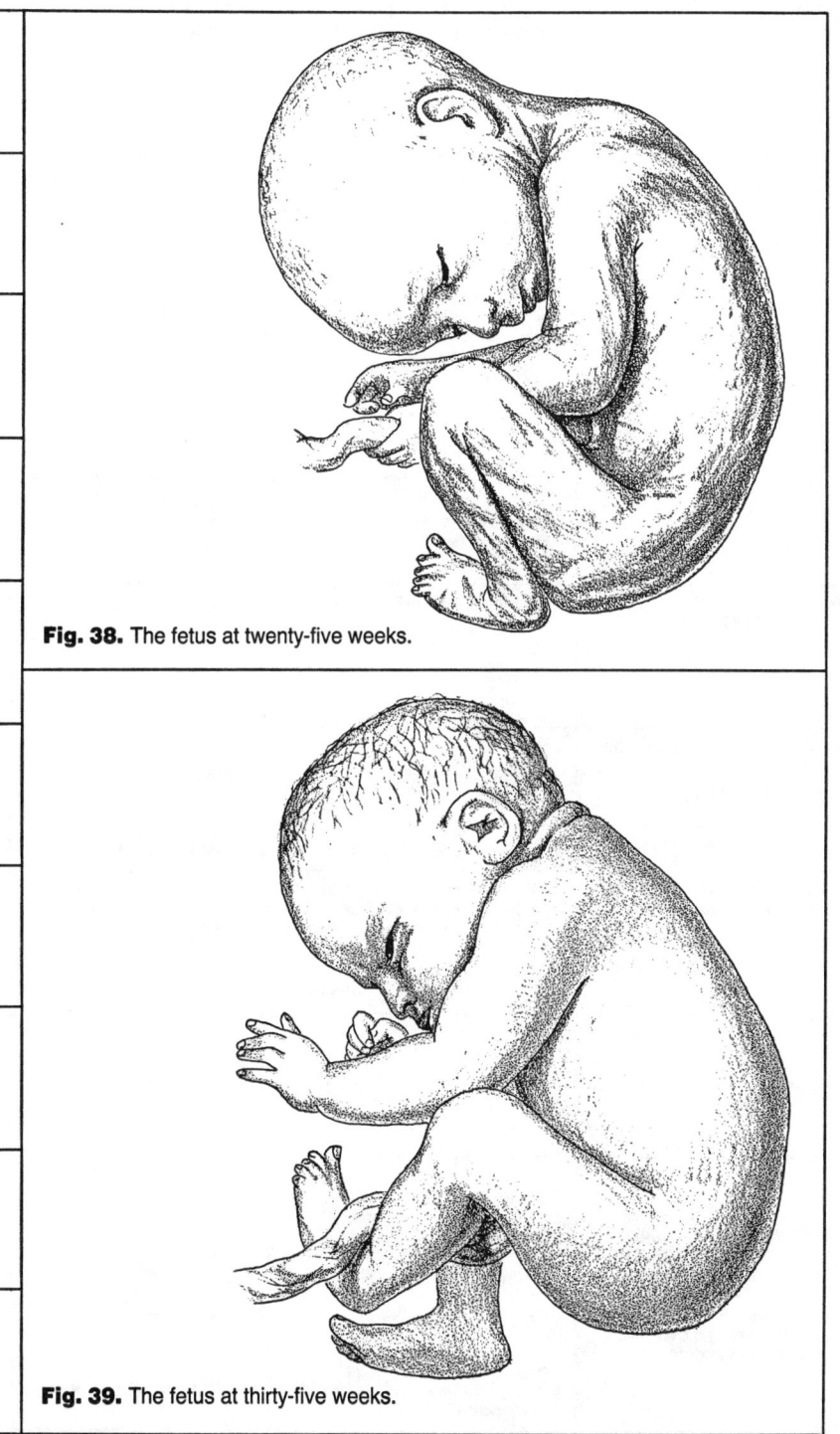

Fig. 38. The fetus at twenty-five weeks.

Fig. 39. The fetus at thirty-five weeks.

WEEK	MOTHER BODY CHANGES OBSERVATIONS	BABY DEVELOPMENT ACTIVITIES
31		• The eyelids, which have been sealed closed, can now open.
32	• From now on, weight gain will average about a pound a week.	• The fetus is about 16 inches long and weighs about 3-1/2 pounds.
33	• Signs of pressure on the pelvic organs are noted, including constipation and frequent urination.	• Most fetuses have moved to a head-down position by this time, although changes in position can occur up to (and during) labor.
34		• In late pregnancy, some light filters into the uterine cavity. The fetus's eyes have been fully developed for several months and will respond to light. Bright light (such as sunshine on the mother's abdomen) causes an increase in fetal movements.
35		• The body appears plump by this time.
36	• The uterus typically is pressing up to the rib cage by now, causing some shortness of breath and heartburn.	• The fetus is about 18 inches long and weighs about 5 pounds.
37	• Uterine contractions have become more noticeable, though still irregular and inconsistent.	• Mild breathing movements, as well as occasional hiccups, occur by this time. Sharp kicks have often diminished by now, due to restriction of movement as the baby grows and fattens. • Muscle tone is good, with arms and legs actively flexing.
38		
39	• During the last two weeks, the height of the uterus may decrease somewhat as the baby's head settles down into the pelvis.	• Fetal weight gain usually stops at about this time, due to aging of the placenta.
40	• Most mothers deliver between 38 and 42 weeks after conception; only 5 percent, however, deliver on their due date.	• Amniotic fluid volume peaks, at about one quart. • The average fetus is about 20 inches long and weighs about 7-1/2 pounds.

APPEARANCE OF GROWING FETUS

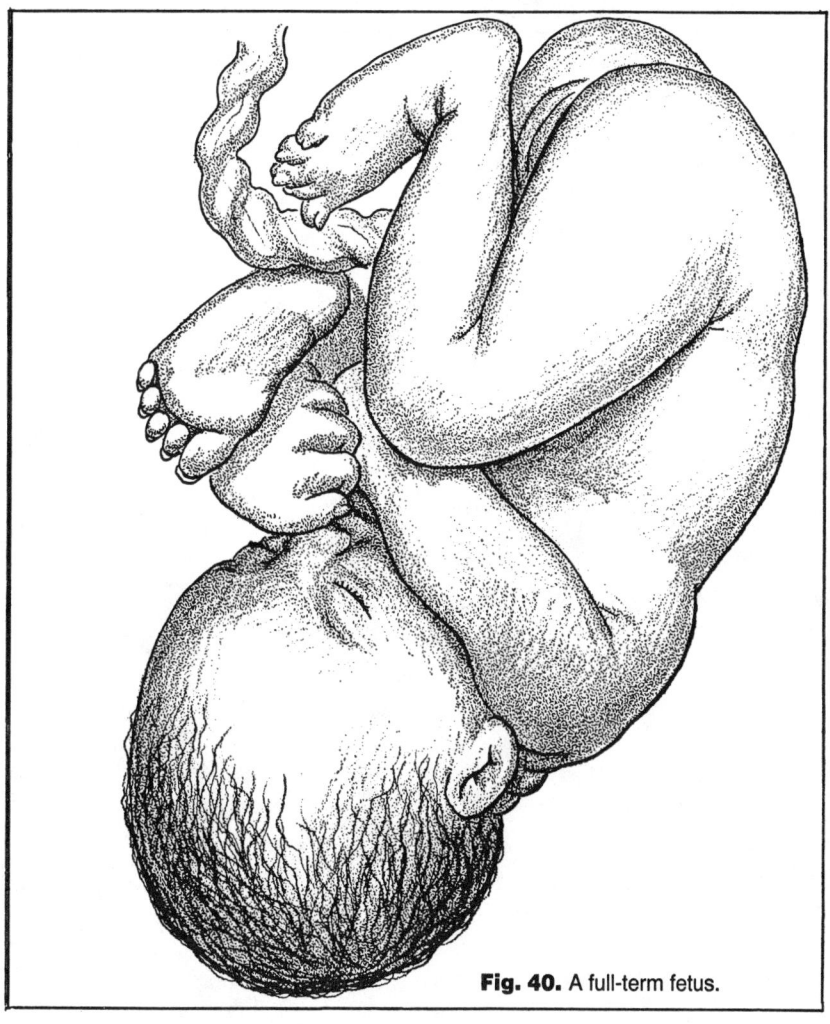

Fig. 40. A full-term fetus.

PART IV

The Last Three Months
27–40 WEEKS

Huge and melon-shaped, the curving bowl of your pregnant abdomen is stretched full with the baby, the enlarged
uterus, heavy and ripe, the life-giving tree of blood vessels
in the placenta and the great sac of water contained in the
membranes. You can reach down and feel your baby and
its outlines under your hands. Wait till you feel a kick and
notice the hard knobs of the little feet. By this time they may
be under your ribs on the left or right side. . . . Your baby
may get hiccups sometimes and you feel a quick knock-
knock-knock or it may be turning its head quickly from side
to side trying to find a lost thumb which it was happily sucking. Its heart beats at about double the rate of your own, at
120 to 160 beats a minute. Now your partner may even be
able to hear this simply by resting his head against your
abdomen.

—Sheila Kitzinger, *The Birth Diary*

Things often seem to slow down during the third trimester.
Growth of your uterus makes moving around more difficult,
and tiredness may be more noticeable. Your thoughts center
more and more on labor and the birth of your new baby.
You'll begin childbirth preparation in earnest now and start
to buy things for the baby.

17 Prenatal Care in Late Pregnancy

As your pregnancy gets further along, the visits to your physician or midwife will follow the general routine of prenatal care described in chapter 5. Your urine, weight, and blood pressure will be checked each time, the size of the uterus will be measured, and the baby's heartbeat will be listened to. Your health-care provider will also ask some questions to learn how you've been feeling. As your pregnancy approaches your due date, there are a few additional things that may be done during your prenatal visits.

Weekly Checkups

In late pregnancy, your health-care provider will ask to see you more and more often, until you are coming in weekly. Changes in the health and positioning of the baby, as well as in your own health, need to be checked more carefully as you approach your due date.

At each visit to your health-care provider, you will be asked about how the baby is moving inside your uterus. Fetal movements provide a day-to-day reminder that the developing baby is alive and growing. These intermittent kicks, bumps, wiggles, and hiccups tend to become less intense in the last few weeks of pregnancy, particularly a day or two before labor begins. They should continue to be noticeable, however, throughout the latter weeks of pregnancy and during labor.

If you do not notice your baby moving, this may be a sign of problems. Your health-care provider may have specific instructions for observing and reporting your baby's movements. If you do not feel your baby move for as long as a day, we recommend that you lie quietly on your side for one hour in the evening and count any movements you feel. If there are three or fewer movements in one hour, call your health-care provider to report this.

During your prenatal visits in late pregnancy, the positioning of the fetus will be checked. By the last few weeks, the baby has often settled down into the position that it will assume during labor. Your physician or midwife will try to figure out whether the head is up or down by feeling the shape of the baby through your abdomen. He or she will also listen with a stethoscope to determine where the placenta is located and to be certain that there aren't two heartbeats (twins!) instead of one.

You may also have a vaginal examination (feeling with one or two fingers in the vagina) to see whether the cervix has begun to soften and thin out (efface). This softening and thinning of the cervix often occurs within a week or so before labor begins. It isn't a very good predictor of when labor will begin, however, because it doesn't happen at the same time in all individuals. For example, it's not unusual for a woman whose cervix is thin and two or three centimeters dilated to spend weeks without going into labor, whereas another with a thick cervix goes into labor within a day. Because vaginal examinations don't really predict when labor is approaching, some health-care providers do not perform them routinely until the fortieth or forty-first week.

If You Pass Your Due Date without Going into Labor

Only about 5 percent of women actually deliver *on* their due date. About 50 percent deliver within 10 days on either side of that date. Quite a few do not go into labor for more than a week beyond their due date.

If you have passed your due date without having your baby, remember that all babies *do* deliver eventually, and almost always within three weeks of the due date. As the days pass, however, it can seem an eternity to wait, bulging uncomfortably, not wanting to plan anything in case labor begins.

Physicians become concerned about a pregnancy when it goes too far beyond 40 weeks, because the chance of complications rises after a pregnancy is more than two weeks late. The reason for this increased complication rate is "aging" of the placenta: it appears that placentas are designed to last exactly 40 weeks and begin to work less efficiently soon afterwards. When a pregnancy goes beyond its due date, the first question is whether the date was correctly calculated. Assuming an accurate due date, physicians and other health-care providers begin to check a woman more frequently as the pregnancy approaches 42 weeks.

If you haven't delivered by the forty-first week (one week past your due date), your health-care provider will do a vaginal examination to determine the baby's position and to look for effacement of the cervix. He or she will discuss with you your sense of the baby's movements, because a baby that is moving well is probably healthy. If there is need for further analysis of the baby's condition, you may be asked to have a fetal activity test or an oxytocin challenge test.

The *fetal activity test* is frequently done in late pregnancy to check the health of the baby and placenta. The basic principle of this test is that a healthy baby moves frequently, and that it briefly increases its heart rate as it moves. The test involves recording the baby's movement while an electronic fetal monitor, attached to your abdomen by a belt, records the baby's heartbeat. A normal fetal activity test requires about four movements with heartbeat acceleration over a 20- or 30-minute period.

If the fetal activity test does not record enough movements or is otherwise abnormal, most physicians then perform an *oxytocin challenge test*. Again, you are connected to a monitor, and the baby's heart rate is recorded. While you are given a drug called oxytocin intravenously to cause mild contractions, the test measures not only how the baby does on its own, but also how it responds to the "challenge" of uterine contractions.

A normal fetal activity test or oxytocin challenge test nearly always indicates that the baby and placenta are healthy, and that they are likely to remain so for at least one week.

If you pass the forty-second week without going into labor, your physician or midwife will check your progress even more closely. The chronology of your pregnancy will be reviewed again, since incorrect estimation of the due date is the most common reason for "late" deliveries. If you appear to be truly beyond 42 weeks, your health-care provider will begin to consider inducing labor.

18 Emotions and Sexuality, 3

For both parents-to-be, the last three months of pregnancy—especially the ninth month—will probably seem the longest. Unfortunately, as the expectant mother grows larger, time appears to gradually slow down. Impatience may be the most prevalent feeling now.

THE EXPECTANT MOTHER

This is the trimester when you will finalize your plans for labor and delivery, complete arrangements about your job, prepare the baby's layette, decide on the baby's name, and take care of all the other details, large and small, that cannot be left to the months ahead. The moment you have been waiting for is almost at hand! Think through your plans carefully—the longer you prepare for the time after the baby's arrival, the more comfortable you'll feel with your decisions. On page 259, you will find a checklist of things you may wish to get done prior to delivery; the checklist of supplies for your baby on page 260 will help you in preparing the baby's layette.

Stress

If you experience some added stress, it's no wonder. You're about to embark on a new phase of your life that will be exciting, but also a little scary. Be sure to take care of your own and your partner's needs along with all of those other matters. In fact, put "you" at the top of your list.

You are likely to be irritated by the comments and questions you'll get: "Haven't you had the baby yet?" . . . "You must be having twins!" . . . "I'm sure it's a boy (or girl)" . . . and on and on. Anticipating such remarks, and keeping a sense of humor, may be your best defense.

Here are some further suggestions for coping with stress:

- **communicate**
- **recognize symptoms of stress**
- **educate yourself about labor and delivery**
- **organize your daily tasks**
- **make time for yourself and get some privacy**
- **get physical release** (exercises, walking, or yoga)
- **give yourself a free day occasionally**

Sexuality

Sex during the last trimester of your pregnancy is *not* forbidden. If you use your imagination, it can be as rewarding as ever. Many couples worry about hurting the baby or starting labor early, but these concerns are generally unfounded. If intercourse is uncomfortable for you or anxiety interferes with your enjoyment, remember that intercourse and making love are not absolutely synonymous. There are many ways for you and your partner to express physical love and support for each other.

There are some circumstances when intercourse is not advisable. For example, if your water has broken, intercourse may cause infection.

Fantasy

Your imagination may be especially vivid during the last trimester, manifesting itself in dreams and fantasy. It's common for women to dream about their babies; dreaming helps your subconscious to cope with the imminent changes. Sometimes the dreams can be strange or unsettling. If you have stressful dreams, fantasies, and worries about your baby, it may help to share them with your partner or support group.

Postpartum Depression

After the baby is born, you probably will feel new stresses; preparing yourself now will make things go more smoothly. Whether it's the first time or the fourth, having a baby will bring about drastic changes in your life. Many of those changes will be wonderful—and overwhelming. *Your* main responsibilities are to your baby, yourself, and your partner. Other demands on your time—visitors, housework, and so on—can wait. If you remember these priorities now and after the baby is born, you are already a step ahead. Forget about everything but the essentials until you've rested and feel ready to take on additional concerns.

You've heard of the "postpartum blues." In fact, about half of new mothers report *some* feelings of depression. (Don't *assume* that you will have them; you may not!) Some of this depression may be tiredness, some may be caused by hormonal changes, and some may be the result of fears and insecurities. Whatever the reasons, it can be helpful to plan now for those first few weeks:

- Get help with housework and childcare—as much as you can afford or can get from relatives and friends.
- Sleep—and relax—whenever you can.
- Limit your activities, and try not to make any major changes in your life.
- Don't have unrealistic expectations about what being a devoted parent means—you shouldn't and can't give yourself 100 percent to your baby.
- Re-establish your relationship with your partner—go out together once in a while. (Be considerate of the father's needs and feelings, too.)
- Above all, enjoy your baby, and remind yourself that the postpartum period is temporary.

THE EXPECTANT FATHER

By now you may be quite used to the idea of being an expectant father, but not quite ready for parenthood. Fortunately, there are some things you can do, and ways you can participate, that will help you feel involved and necessary (which you are):

- Attend childbirth education classes with your partner. Help her practice.
- Buy things for the baby.
- Set up the nursery.
- Support your partner and yourself emotionally and mentally.
- Support your partner physically. She will need more help around the house as she gets larger and tires more easily. Massage is a great way to ease tension and cramps.

You may find yourself worrying about your wife's safety and health during labor and delivery; that is a natural concern. Learning about the process of childbirth and talking to fathers who have been through a birth can be very helpful. There will be some blood, varying degrees of pain, and some intense emotional experiences ahead. The best thing you can do is to be prepared.

You may find yourself fantasizing and worrying about what kind of father you will be. That, too, is natural, and a good way to prepare yourself.

While it is probably safe to continue to make love throughout pregnancy, lovemaking during the final weeks can be a problem. Be creative and also sensitive to your partner's comfort. There are ways of touching and showing affection, such as massage, kissing, and hugging, that can take the place of intercourse during these last weeks.

19 About Labor and Delivery

To be born, a baby must squeeze through a narrow and irregularly shaped passageway. For the baby to make its way out, the passageway needs to stretch, and the baby needs to twist and turn. Most babies do this in a standard way (the normal vaginal delivery), but a large number of variations can occur. Here we will describe what happens in normal labor and delivery. In the next chapter, we will discuss some of the more common variations and complications.

How Your Body Changes to Allow Your Baby to Be Born

A narrow pathway from inside the uterus to outside your body is present throughout pregnancy. This natural channel is sealed shut by mucous in the cervix and a wall of thin membrane called the amniotic sac ("bag of waters"). During labor, the pathway through the cervix widens, and the baby's head and body slowly squeeze through a bony and muscular passageway. The specific barriers that hold the baby in are the pelvic bones, the cervix, the walls of the vagina, and the perineal muscles (see fig. 41).

The pelvic bones are shaped to form a short funnel that is slightly wider at the top than at the bottom. Because the pelvis has an irregular shape, the baby's head must turn during its passage to the outside. Pelvic bones come in different sizes and shapes in different women. These variations in bone structure, as well as differences in the size and positioning of the baby, provide much of the explanation for what makes some labors more difficult than others.

The cervix is a round knot of elastic tissue and muscle at the

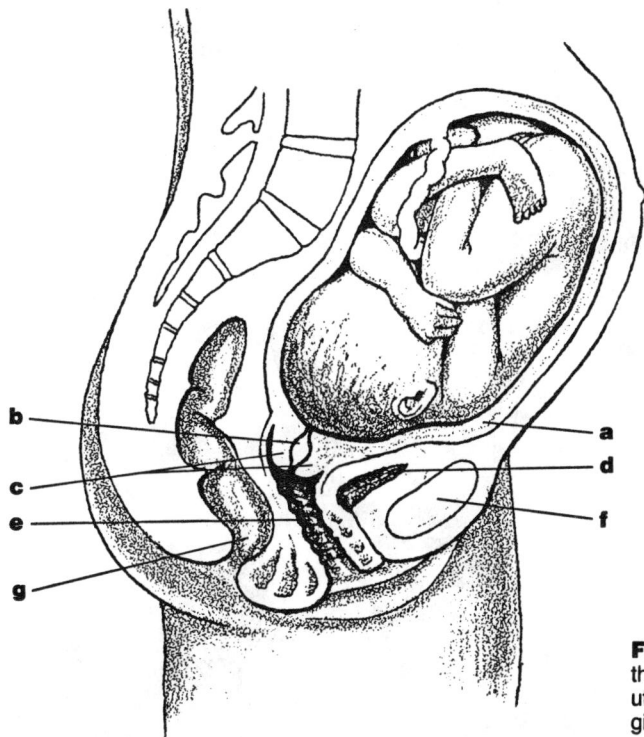

Fig. 41. Cross section of a woman's pelvis, showing the major structures related to childbirth: (a) lower uterus, (b) mucous plug, (c) cervix, (d) bladder, (e) vagina, (f) pubic bone, (g) rectum.

bottom of the uterus that forms a tight closure similar to a purse string. The cervix is approximately one inch (two or three centimeters) long throughout most of pregnancy. During labor, it shortens and thins out (effaces) and then opens (dilates) so that the baby's head and body can leave the uterus (see fig. 42).

The walls of the vagina are muscular and elastic. They contain many folds that enable them to stretch to accommodate the baby's passage. As the baby is pushed lower and lower, the vagina's stretchy walls slowly slide around the baby's head and body.

The muscles of the pelvic floor (perineum) come last. They must be relaxed and stretched during the final phase of labor. These muscles form a kind of sling that holds the vagina closed. They are located under and roughly parallel to your labia and extend from the pubic bone to your tailbone, encircling the anus and vagina (see fig. 9, on page 55). These muscles are what you tighten up when you hold your urine in or do Kegel exercises. They form the final barrier to the baby's birth.

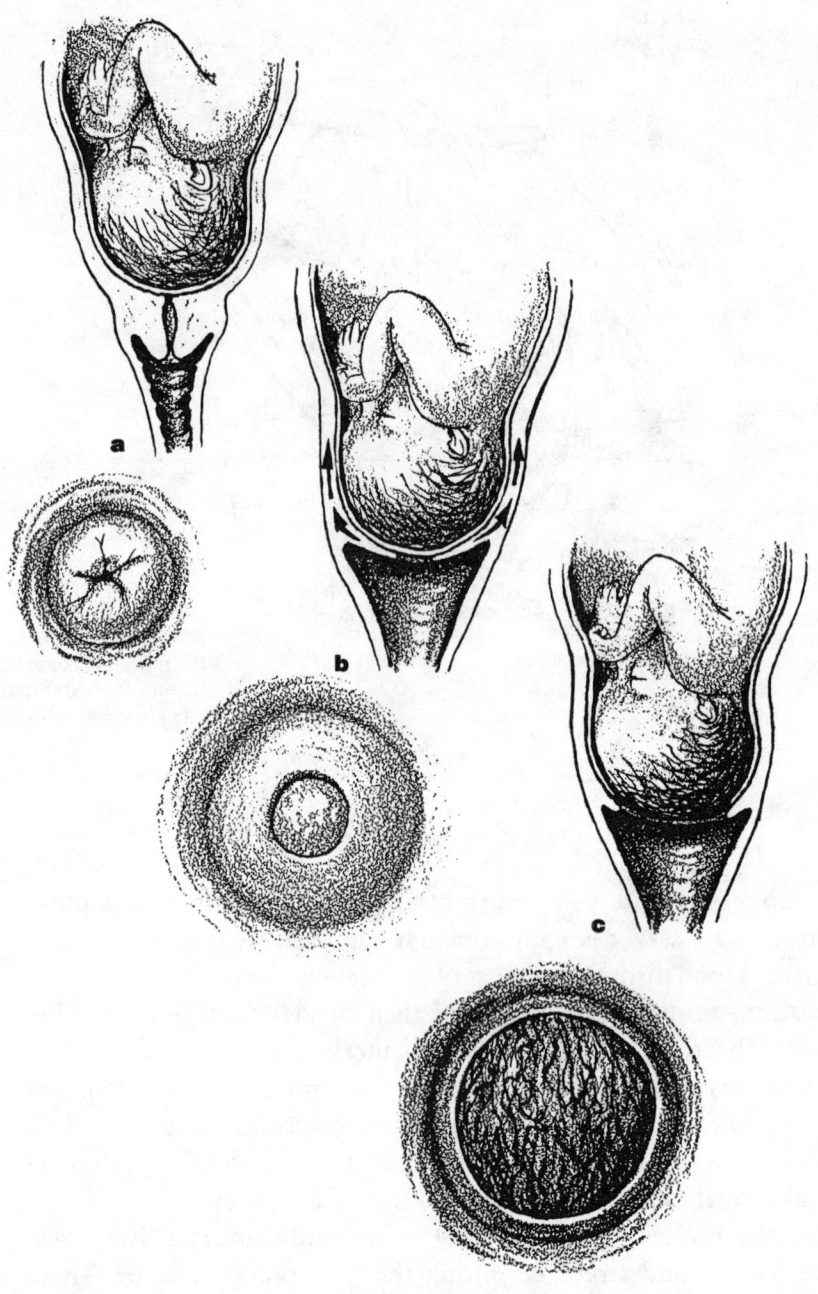

Fig. 42. How the cervix changes during labor: (a) cervix prior to labor, (b) appearance after cervix has effaced fully and dilated to 1½ centimeters, (c) appearance after cervix is dilated eight centimeters. The hair on the baby's head is visible through the open cervix.

How a Baby Is Born

No one knows exactly why labor occurs when it does or what gets labor started; it's different for each individual. The beginning of labor has something to do with a hormone called oxytocin, which is made in the pituitary gland. (Doctors use oxytocin to induce labor.) Oxytocin will not start labor, however, unless the uterus is ready.

Labor itself consists of regular contractions (tightening) of the muscles of the uterus. The contractions cause the cervix to thin out and dilate (open) and cause the baby to be pushed lower into the pelvis and toward the vagina. The muscles of the uterus are among the strongest muscles in the human body; so the contractions are very intense.

The first thing that happens in most labors is that the baby's head settles down into the pelvis. This process is called engagement. In most women who have not had a baby, engagement occurs two or three weeks prior to labor. In women who have previously had a child, engagement usually doesn't occur until labor begins. Engagement leads to a feeling of being able to breathe easier ("lightening"), and the bulge of the uterus becomes noticeably lower in the abdomen.

At about the same time, the cervix begins to thin out from a length of two or three centimeters to only a few millimeters. This thinning of the cervix is called effacement and is produced by the muscular contractions of the uterus. As the uterus contracts, it pulls the cervix up into the wall of the uterus itself, causing it to appear to thin out and gradually disappear. Health-care providers describe the process of effacement as a percentage. Thus, "50 percent effaced" implies that the cervix has progressed halfway from being three centimeters long to being paper thin (see fig. 42).

Once the cervix has effaced, it then begins to dilate. This process is referred to as dilation or dilatation. (The word dilatation is ungrammatical but is deeply ingrained in the medical profession; so, you will very likely hear it used.) Dilation itself is really just a continuation of effacement. Once the contractions of the uterine muscles have pulled the cervix up into the wall of the uterus, they continue to pull until the hole enlarges more and more. Eventually, the cervix has opened up to a diameter of about 10 centimeters (four inches), which is wide enough to permit the passage of the baby's head.

At the same time the cervix is dilating, the contractions of the uterus are slowly pushing the baby through the funnel-shaped pelvic bones. Just how fast a baby descends through the pelvis varies from person to person. The narrowest portion of the pelvis is an area that contains two small bumps of bone, called the ischial spines, which are used as a landmark by doctors and midwives. Your health-care provider will examine you during labor to determine the position of the top of the baby's head relative to the ischial spines. This relative position is called the baby's "station" (fig. 43). A baby that is at a station of −1 has the top of its head one centimeter above the ischial spines. During labor, the baby's head progresses from approximately −3 through station 0 (when the top of the head is even with the spines) to a +3 station. By the time a +3 station is reached, the baby's head can be seen pushing out from between the bulging labia, and delivery is generally only minutes away.

While descending through the pelvis, the head must also rotate 90 degrees, because the top of the pelvis has a different shape than the bottom of the pelvis. In most women (a few pelvises are shaped differently), the baby's head enters the pelvis facing to one side and comes out facing frontwards or backwards. Most commonly, the

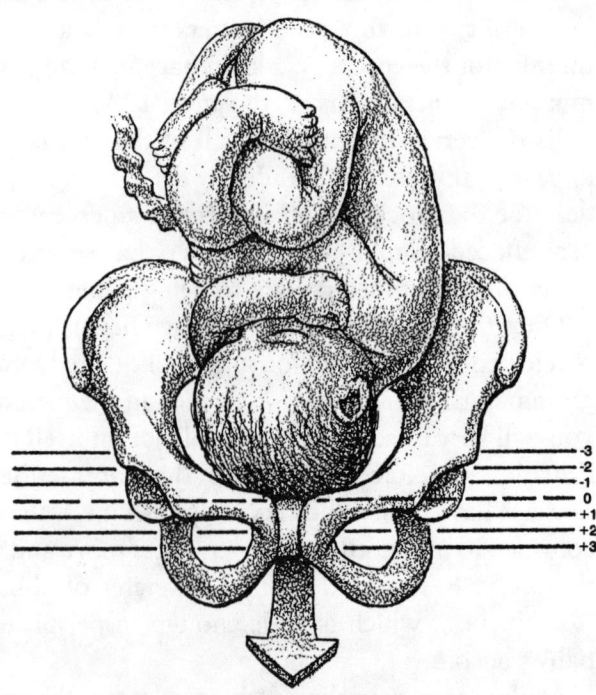

Fig. 43. Schematic diagram of the pelvic bones, showing how the position of the baby's head, called the "station," is measured. Station zero indicates that the top of the baby's head is even with the ischial spines.

baby emerges with the top of its head sliding under the mother's pubic bone and the face turned toward the mother's anus.

The whole process of labor is accompanied by contractions of the uterus ("labor pains"). During these contractions, the best thing you can do is relax your muscles. Much of childbirth education (such as Lamaze classes) involves teaching you to control the discomfort of labor. In addition, medication is often given to help. Later, you will aid the uterine contractions by using your own abdominal muscles to help push the baby down through the pelvis and out the vagina.

The final barrier, the muscles of the perineum, begins bulging when the head is at +3 station. Slowly, the head of the baby thins and stretches the perineal muscles until they form an opening wide enough for the baby to be born. Learning to relax these muscles by doing Kegel exercises will help in this phase of labor. If it appears that the muscles are not stretching enough to permit birth of the head, the physician or midwife will make a cut through some of the perineal muscles. This cut is called an episiotomy.

The Stages of Labor and Delivery

Every woman has contractions of the uterus for months prior to going into labor. These contractions are called Braxton Hicks, or false labor, contractions. Some women are aware of these contractions, whereas others are not. The contractions themselves are irregular, sometimes strong, and sometimes very mild. When they are strong and occur close together, they can be mistaken for labor. (Note: Labor can begin before your due date, and if this happens you should contact your health-care provider right away. See page 147 for a discussion of premature labor.) Braxton Hicks contractions are important in developing the tone and strength of the uterus. In addition, they can accomplish some thinning and dilating of the cervix. Thus, by the time labor begins, the cervix is often about 50 percent effaced and one or two centimeters dilated.

Labor itself has three stages (see table 5). The *first stage*, which is by far the longest, consists of the time that it takes to efface and dilate the cervix. It lasts an average of 10 to 14 hours for the first baby; in subsequent labors, it tends to shorten. The *second stage* consists of active pushing with the abdominal muscles and lasts an hour or two on the average. At the end of the second stage, the baby is born. The *third stage* consists of waiting for the placenta to come out.

Table 5. The Stages of Labor and Delivery

Stage	Contractions	Changes in cervix	Average duration	
			First pregnancy	Subsequent labors
Prelabor	Irregular and mild	Very minimal; some efface-ment occurs	Weeks	Weeks
First stage				
Latent phase	Regular; mild to moderate; progressing from far apart to every 5–10 minutes	Effacement and dilation to 3 centimeters	5–7 hours	3–5 hours
Active phase	Regular; moderate to severe; every 3–5 minutes	Dilation from 3–8 centimeters	5 hours	3 hours
Transition	Regular and intense, often associated with shivering and nausea/vomiting; every 2–3 minutes	Dilation from 8–10 centimeters	1 hour	½ hour
Second stage (pushing)	Quite intense; every 2–4 minutes	Descent of head; delivery of the baby	60–90 minutes	20–30 minutes
Third stage (delivery of the placenta)	Few, relatively mild	Begins to contract slightly	5–20 minutes	5–20 minutes

The first stage, constituting the majority of the time spent in labor, can be further divided into three phases: *latent phase*, *active phase*, and *transition*.

Latent Phase

During latent phase—the first six to eight hours of labor—contractions are usually relatively mild. By the end of the phase, the cervix will have effaced almost completely and dilated two or three centimeters. Often, the earliest contractions will not be noticed, particularly if you happen to be asleep or very busy.

Sometime during latent phase, however, you will probably become aware that you are having regular contractions. You will call or awaken your partner, time the contractions, and decide that labor has indeed begun. After a number of hours—it varies widely—the labor will intensify so that the contractions are closer together, coming regularly every five minutes or so. This indicates that you are entering active phase.

Active Phase

Once the cervix dilates to about three centimeters, contractions become stronger, and labor is said to have entered active phase. This phase is usually quite intense, and some kind of pain relief in the form of controlled breathing, self-hypnosis, massage, and/or medication is generally needed. Because contractions clearly intensify as active phase begins, this is often the time when a woman in labor wants to go to the hospital.

Active phase averages five hours during first labors, and tends to shorten each additional time a woman goes through labor. Active phase ends when the cervix is dilated to eight or nine centimeters.

Transition

As the cervix reaches eight or nine centimeters, the contractions intensify even more, coming every two or three minutes. This transition phase generally lasts between half an hour and two hours, ending when the cervix is completely dilated. For many women, it is the most difficult part of labor. The intense contractions are often accompanied by nausea, vomiting, shivering, and irritability. It is during this time that a partner or coach, and the techniques learned in childbirth education classes, can be particularly valuable.

In addition, if the head is beginning to descend, you may become aware of a desire to try to push the baby out with your abdominal muscles. This urge to push needs to be resisted until the cervix is completely dilated, since pushing against an incompletely dilated cervix may injure the cervix. Pushing when the cervix is not completely dilated is like driving a car through a gate that is not completely open. The gate (cervix) will stop your progress until it is opened and may be injured, and bleed, if it is forced.

The Second Stage of Labor: Pushing

Finally, the cervix is fully dilated, and it is time to push. The second stage of labor has now begun. Usually, this comes as a relief, because active pushing tends to feel better than holding back and trying to relax during contractions. Some people say pushing is like straining to have a bowel movement, only much harder; others say it's different because you push from higher up and must relax your bottom. When properly instructed, however, most women have little trouble learning to push effectively in labor.

Pushing gradually brings the baby's head down. This may take a few minutes or as long as a couple of hours, but eventually the pelvic floor muscles visibly bulge with each push. At this time, you may feel an intense burning sensation, which indicates that the perineal muscles are stretching. In spite of this discomfort, it is important to try to keep those muscles relaxed and to continue pushing. An episiotomy might be made at this point, and the baby's head finally emerges.

Birth of the Baby

As soon as the baby's head slides through the labia, you will be asked to stop pushing for a moment so the doctor or midwife can suck mucous and fluid out of the baby's nostrils and mouth. This procedure makes it easier for the baby to take its first breath. The doctor or midwife then checks to see if the umbilical cord is wrapped around the baby's neck, freeing the cord if it is. Then, the shoulders and body are delivered. During this time, some pushing is also helpful, and your doctor or midwife will let you know when to do so. The baby begins to breathe, the umbilical cord is clamped and cut, and a new person enters the world.

Hospital Routines during Labor

If you plan to deliver in a hospital, it will be helpful for you to understand and anticipate the routines and personnel you will encounter there. Hospitals vary in their policies, but the trend overall is for more flexibility, fewer "routine" interventions, and for greater consideration of labor as a natural event than in years past.

In the hospital, you will encounter several staff members. These may include:

● **Nursing staff.** They will check on the progress of your labor by frequently taking your blood pressure and pulse, listening to the baby's heartbeat, observing your contractions, and carrying out certain special procedures (such as electronic monitoring) if needed. Nurses often seek to improve your comfort by offering ice water, rubbing your back, showing you how to relax during contractions, making sure you empty your bladder, and so on.

● **Physicians (and midwives).** In general, the more difficult your labor is, or the more concerned your physician is about possible complications of labor and delivery, the more personal attention he or she will give. Midwives tend to spend more time in the labor room, providing support during labor. If

you have a good support person and your labor is going well, your physician
or midwife will probably check on you periodically by talking with you and the
nurses, and by examining the baby's progress.

● **Administrative staff.** On admission, you will need to have certain
hospital paperwork completed for billing purposes. Often, this can be
completed in advance by pre-registering. (We recommend you find out about
pre-registration at your hospital and complete as much of the paperwork as
you can beforehand.) Other administrative paperwork involves identifying the
baby and completing the birth certificate. Thus, it is rare not to encounter one
or more administrative staff while in the hospital.

● **Cleaning staff.** Keeping the hospital spotless is an important and
continuing task. However, if cleaning staff, repairmen, or maintenance
personnel enter your room while you are in labor, you should not hesitate to
ask them to leave.

On admission to the hospital, you will probably be taken to an
admitting room in the labor area. There, you will be asked to give
a urine specimen, your baby's heartbeat will be listened to, and
someone (usually a nurse) will ask questions about your labor. You
will be examined by a physician, midwife, or nurse to determine
if, indeed, you are in labor—and, if so, how far the labor has
progressed.

Assuming you are in labor and progressing normally, you will
then be moved to a labor room. Labor rooms vary widely. Some
are designed to accommodate several women at a time, usually on
hospital stretchers, separated by thin curtains. This type of arrangement makes medical and nursing observations easier but sacrifices much privacy and comfort. At the other extreme are "home-
style" labor rooms, with beds, rocking chairs, radio or television,
and privacy. A few home-style rooms have a birthing chair, a kind
of seat specially designed to be comfortable when used during
pushing and giving birth. Other home-style rooms have large pillows or a warm whirlpool to enhance comfort during labor. Since
there is such variation in labor rooms, you should find out in advance what facilities are available at your hospital and whether you
have some choice.

When your labor is nearly complete and the baby is about to be
born, you may be moved to a delivery room. All hospital delivery
rooms include operating room lights, a delivery table (with stir-
rups for your feet), and a large amount of medical equipment.
These rooms are designed to accommodate any possible medical
need, including general anesthesia, caesarean section, and stabili-
zation of an ill baby. For the average delivery, such sophisticated

technology is unnecessary, however. Therefore, many hospitals permit you to give birth in a home-style labor room or some similar setting (such as a birthing center). Ask in advance about your options.

Many questions may occur to you about the way your health-care provider will manage your labor and delivery. Often, there will be choices available to you and your health-care provider, and these should be discussed in advance whenever possible.

20 Variations and Complications in Labor and Delivery

In the previous chapter, we went over the details of the "typical" labor and delivery. When it comes to individuals, though, unpredictability seems to be the rule. The odds are pretty good that something will happen to make your childbirth experience different than we've outlined so far. The variations in the way childbirth occurs can range from differences in obstetric technique (such as episiotomy) to serious complications for the mother or baby. Here we will discuss some of the problems related to childbirth and tell you about certain medical procedures designed to handle complications.

Premature Labor

Premature labor is defined as going into labor before you are 37 or 38 weeks pregnant. It increases the likelihood of medical complications for the baby, particularly breathing problems and the need for resuscitation or intensive care. Therefore, it is important to be aware of the signs of premature labor so you can report them to your health-care provider if they occur.

We don't know why labor begins early in some pregnancies. There are a number of things that make premature labor more likely, including previous premature labor, severe illness in the mother, certain complications of pregnancy, and a stressful living situation.

More important than knowing these risk factors is for you to be aware of the signs of premature labor:

- **menstrual-like cramps or a dull backache**
- **abdominal cramping, with or without diarrhea**
- **uterine contractions that are regular and ten minutes apart or less** (they do *not* have to be painful)
- **pressure low down in the abdomen, felt as a heaviness or like the baby pushing down**
- **watery discharge or a gush of fluid from the vagina**

If you have signs of premature labor, we recommend that you lie down on your side for one hour. While resting, drink two or three glasses of water or juice. Often, resting and drinking fluids will make the symptoms of premature labor subside. If they do not go away in an hour, however, you should call your health-care provider.

If you do go into labor prematurely, you will need to be hospitalized under a physician's care. Your physician will ask you to rest in bed on your side. Your contractions will be observed and recorded using an electronic monitor (see below). Your physician will discuss with you the benefits and risks of stopping labor and the likelihood of complications for the baby. He or she may then decide to use a medication to try to stop the labor. Unfortunately, medicines for halting premature labor are not always successful. If labor continues, or if your physician decides that it is best not to try to stop it, your labor will be monitored electronically and you will deliver in a room equipped to stabilize ill newborns. A pediatrician will probably be present to take care of the baby.

Caesarean Section

Caesarean section (named after Julius Caesar, who was reportedly born by this method) is the surgical removal of the baby through an incision in the mother's abdomen. In skilled hands, it is quite safe for the baby; in fact, it is probably safer than vaginal delivery for some conditions. Its major drawback is its risk to the health of the mother, not to the baby.

Caesarean section requires anesthesia and opening up the abdomen, both of which have small but significant complication rates. The decision to deliver by caesarean section is, therefore, something to be carefully considered and discussed openly, if time allows. Caesarean section should not be considered a failure of natural childbirth but rather an alternative method of having a baby that is used when needed.

Bleeding before or during Labor

A small amount of blood and mucous ("bloody show") often appears in the vagina around the time labor begins. It is unusual, however, to have more than a couple of tablespoons of bleeding in late pregnancy or during labor. Considerable bleeding can occur immediately after birth, as the placenta separates from the uterus. However, bleeding at any time in the third trimester or before birth can signify a serious threat to the baby. One such problem is *abruption of the placenta*, in which the placenta begins to separate from the uterus early. Another reason for major bleeding late in pregnancy is *placenta previa*, meaning that the placenta is located between the baby and the birth canal. Since both of these conditions are potentially quite serious, report any bleeding greater than two tablespoons to your health-care provider.

Monitoring

Over the past decade, electronic recording of the baby's heartbeat and of uterine contractions in labor has become quite popular, and in many places, routine. This minute-by-minute information provides far more detailed data on how the baby is doing and how the labor is progressing than does listening periodically with a stethoscope. It has disadvantages, however: it prevents the woman from moving about freely and can be used as a poor substitute for personal care by doctors and nurses. In addition, there is much about monitoring that is unknown, and the significance of subtle changes in the baby's heart rate has not been determined.

The most common form of monitoring involves attaching two wires to the woman in labor. Each of the wires is attached either *externally* (on your abdomen) or *internally* (inside the vagina). One wire, which can be attached to a belt around your belly or directly to the baby's head, records the baby's heartbeat. The other wire, which can be attached to a separate belt around your abdomen or slid in a tube past the baby's head directly into the uterus, measures your contractions. Both are attached to a machine that records the information on special graph paper.

Rupture of Membranes before Labor Starts

The uterus is tightly sealed by a thin, tough membrane that is somewhat like cellophane. This membrane holds in the amniotic fluid (called "the water") and keeps out bacteria. Because it is pulled on as the cervix dilates, this membrane usually breaks (ruptures) sometime during labor. When this happens, amniotic fluid comes out—sometimes in a trickle, sometimes in a gush.

In around 10 percent of pregnancies, the membranes rupture (the water "breaks") before labor starts. If this happens, the protective barrier against infection is broken, posing a serious threat to the baby. Within as little as 24 hours after rupture, infection can develop in the uterus. For this reason, health-care providers will try to get labor started if it doesn't begin on its own. Fortunately, labor often begins on its own soon after the membranes rupture.

In the event your water breaks, notify your physician or midwife at once. If you are already in labor, you should be examined to be certain the gush of fluid did not carry part of the baby's umbilical cord into the cervical opening. If you are not in labor, your health-care provider will want to confirm that amniotic fluid is leaking, check the baby's position, and observe you for signs of labor.

If your membranes rupture and you are many weeks premature, it may be safest to keep the baby inside the uterus. In that situation, your health-care provider will watch closely for signs of infection and hope that the leak closes.

Rapid Labor

Some women are blessed with unusually rapid labors, often going to full dilation of the cervix within a few hours. There are potential complications, including an increased tendency for the vagina to tear and a greater likelihood of bleeding from the uterus after delivery. In general, however, rapid labor is a welcome event.

Slow Labor

Although nearly everyone would be happy to have a shorter labor, some labors progress particularly slowly. Often, when this happens, there is a tight fit between the baby and the pelvis, and sometimes a caesarean section is needed. On other occasions, labor is slow due to the mother being excessively tired, to medications given as pain relief, or to contractions of the uterus that are not particularly effective. If your labor is progressing slowly, your physician or midwife will attempt to decide what the problem is and to help improve your labor. If your contractions are not strong enough, nipple stimulation or oxytocin may be used to strengthen them (see below).

Induced Labor

There are four general reasons why your labor may be artificially induced: if your water breaks and labor fails to begin, if your pregnancy goes beyond 42 weeks, if there is a medical problem that threatens your own or your baby's health and for which the treatment is delivery, and if you are in labor but the contractions are not strong enough. The last situation mentioned is referred to as *augmentation*, because the labor is only being assisted, not started.

To induce or augment labor, physicians use a drug called oxytocin, which is a natural substance your body produces to bring on labor and to stimulate milk production. Rubbing your breasts releases some oxytocin, and nipple stimulation (only a few health-care providers try this) can sometimes make the use of medication unnecessary. If you do receive oxytocin, you will be attached by intravenous line to a special pump that injects the medicine at a specified rate. The oxytocin is begun in a low dose and gradually increased until labor contractions develop. Because the contractions must be measured, you will be attached to an electronic monitor.

Induced labor tends to be shorter than natural labor. The contractions are generally stronger and more painful, however. Another drawback is that the monitoring limits your ability to move around.

Unusually Painful Labor

It's hard to explain why some labors are more painful than others. Some women have higher pain tolerances than others, but that does not really explain the variation we see. In fact, how much discomfort labor causes seems to have more to do with the individual labor itself rather than with pain tolerance. Occasionally, a labor will be particularly painful, even during false labor or the earliest stages. When this happens, medication becomes essential to help the mother through labor. (See chapter 21 for a discussion of the management of pain in labor.)

Difficulty with Pushing

Some women go through the first stage of labor quite well and dilate to 10 centimeters, only to have difficulty with pushing. The cause may be tiredness or drugs used for pain relief. Pushing sometimes goes slowly because the baby needs to make some accommodation before its head can continue down the birth canal. Specifically, the head may need to rotate, or the bones of the head may compress and overlap slightly (a safe, natural method of decreasing the size of the baby's head called molding).

Often, good coaching can overcome difficulties with pushing. Sometimes, even the best efforts at pushing fail to deliver the baby. If this happens, delivery by forceps or vacuum extractor may be necessary; or, if the baby's head has not come down far enough, a caesarean section may be needed.

Forceps Delivery and Vacuum Extraction

When pushing brings the baby partway down the birth canal but cannot complete the delivery, forceps delivery or vacuum extraction may be used. Both techniques replace or assist the mother's pushing by putting traction on the baby's head. (In other words, instruments are used to gently pull the baby free.) The forceps is a device something like specialized tweezers or tongs. Shaped to fit the curve of a baby's head, the two arms of the forceps are put on one side at a time and then locked together. The vacuum extractor is a round metal or plastic cup held by a vacuum to the top of the baby's head.

These methods sound (and look) somewhat frightening. Both have been used for many years, however, and are generally quite safe for the baby. In fact, forceps protect the baby's head so well that they are often used to prevent injury when premature infants (which have delicate heads) are born.

When forceps and vacuum extraction are used, doctors usually perform an episiotomy. Lacerations of the vagina are also more common when these instruments are used. The other common complications result from the firmness with which the baby must be pulled. Forceps can leave mild bruises or pressure marks on the side of the baby's head. After delivery by vacuum extractor, swelling of the baby's scalp is common. All these marks are usually gone within a few days.

Sudden Slowing of the Baby's Heartbeat

When you are in labor, nurses and doctors will listen to your baby's heartbeat frequently. You may also be attached to a monitoring device that continuously records the baby's heartbeat. Slowing of the heartbeat can be a sign that the baby is having difficulty during labor. This slowing can occur in a number of patterns: some are normal; others definitely indicate problems. If your baby's heartbeat slows, you may be asked to move to a different side or up on your knees, because pressure on the umbilical cord can affect the heartbeat and is relieved by changes in position. You may also be given oxygen, or you may be advised to stop pushing temporarily. These simple measures often help the baby recover from the stress of labor. Occasionally, when the baby's heartbeat continues to be slow despite these maneuvers, rapid delivery by forceps, vacuum extractor, or caesarean section is necessary.

Preeclampsia (Toxemia)

Preeclampsia (also called toxemia) is a relatively uncommon disease in which high blood pressure and kidney problems develop. It occurs only in pregnancy, usually in the last few weeks, and goes away entirely after the baby is born. It tends to worsen rapidly, not improving until birth. When severe, it can lead to seizures, kidney failure, and heart problems in the mother, and death of the baby can result.

Early signs of preeclampsia include sudden weight gain, swelling of the face and hands, and a rise in blood pressure. Other signs, which usually occur later, are dizziness, severe headache, and spots in front of the eyes.

If you develop mild preeclampsia, it can often be alleviated by lying in bed. More severe preeclampsia requires hospitalization and medication to treat the high blood pressure. Sometimes labor is induced to prevent the problem from worsening. Because high blood pressure can cause early "aging" of the placenta, the labor of a woman with preeclampsia should always be monitored.

Lacerations and Episiotomy

As the baby is delivered, the head or shoulders may tear the cervix, vagina, labia, or perineum. These lacerations can range from a tiny one to a large tear that extends all the way to the rectum. Many factors can result in big lacerations, including a large baby, an unusually rapid delivery, or use of the forceps or vacuum extractor.

Lacerations occurring during delivery can be difficult to stitch together and may occur in especially sensitive places, such as around the urethral opening, where your urine comes out. To avoid these lacerations, physicians came up with the idea of doing a cut below the vagina, which is called an episiotomy. Besides preventing lacerations, an episiotomy can shorten the time a woman has to push in labor, which can be desirable in some situations. Some physicians regularly do episiotomies, but most midwives and physicians wait until it appears that the baby's head will cause a laceration before doing one. If you have particular feelings about an episiotomy, you may wish to speak with your health-care provider about this beforehand.

Meconium in the Amniotic Fluid

If the baby moves its bowels before it is born, it fouls the amniotic fluid, which turns brown or yellowish and sometimes thickens in consistency. The bowel movement is called meconium.

Amniotic fluid that contains meconium is extremely irritating to a newborn's lungs. If much gets into the lungs when a baby first breathes, serious pneumonia can result. Therefore, any baby that has meconium in its amniotic fluid is suctioned particularly carefully during birth to remove as much fluid as possible before it takes its first breath.

Infant Resuscitation

The passage from inside the uterus to the outside is statistically the most dangerous time in a person's life. What a task it is, fitting through such a tight space, and then adjusting to breathing and functioning independently! It's not surprising, therefore, that some babies have initial difficulty breathing on their own. Babies who have trouble breathing immediately after birth require some kind of help, and this is termed resuscitation. It may vary from something as mild as a slap on the back or a vigorous rubdown to oxygen treatment and sophisticated drugs, depending on how severe the problem is.

Most babies respond rapidly and well to resuscitation measures and are normal afterwards. A few require intensive care for vary-

ing periods of time. Those that cannot be successfully revived or
are born dead are termed stillborn.

Stillbirth

A surprising number (about 1 percent) of babies die within a few
days before labor begins, or during labor and delivery itself. These
babies are termed stillbirths.

The cause of death sometimes cannot be explained. Much of the
technology that has developed in obstetrics over the past decades,
such as electronic monitoring, fetal activity tests, and the increased
rate of caesarean sections, has come about in order to discover and
treat problems before a stillbirth occurs. Sometimes the best of
efforts are not successful, however. When a stillbirth happens, physicians and other health professionals attempt to help a couple
cope with the unfortunate event.

Breech Presentation

In about 5 percent of deliveries, the baby is turned rump first instead of head first. This situation is called breech presentation. Because the head has to come out last instead of first, certain problems
may result. The head is the largest part of the baby's body, and after
the rest of the body has emerged, it can have difficulty fitting
through the pelvis. As the head is coming out, the umbilical cord is
already halfway out, and blood flow may then not be good during
delivery of the head. In addition, delivery of the head requires
some traction (gentle pulling), which may cause injury to the nerves
in the baby's neck. If the head is difficult to fit through the pelvis, a
forceps delivery may be necessary.

For these reasons, vaginal delivery of breech babies has a higher
complication rate than delivery of babies that are positioned head
first. If your baby is found in breech position when labor begins,
your doctor will want to consider the merits of a caesarean delivery. The decision will depend on whether you have had babies before, on the size of the baby, on the size of your pelvic opening, and
on the position of the baby's legs in the uterus.

Twins

Giving birth to twins has more than twice the chance of complications than the delivery of one child. When a woman has two babies

in her uterus, each is usually smaller than a single baby would be; thus they are less likely to have problems fitting through the pelvis. By being smaller, however, twins are more likely to have breathing difficulties after birth. In addition, either twin may be positioned head first or breech, and often after delivery of the first twin there is a limited time for the second to get into position. Because the positioning of twins is often not ideal for vaginal delivery, many twins are delivered by caesarean section.

Malformations (Birth Defects)

Around 5 percent of babies are born with some kind of abnormality. The most common birth defects are probably an extra finger or toe and certain birthmarks on the skin. More serious problems with the baby occur less often (1 or 2 percent of the time) and can rarely be anticipated.

If your baby is malformed, it will almost certainly come as a shock. At a time when energy is often depleted, you will have to learn specific information about your baby's condition. You will need support and patience from your partner, family, and health-care provider.

Often, a malformation seems worse when you first learn about it than it turns out to be in the long run. Remarkable advances in surgery and medical treatment have made many severe birth defects treatable. Nevertheless, if you are faced with this un-expected event, you will need—and should seek—comforting and encouragement.

Retained Placenta

After the baby is delivered, the placenta usually separates and comes out of the uterus within 30 minutes. Occasionally, the placenta just doesn't seem to feel like letting go, which can cause bleeding by preventing the uterus from tightening up. When this happens, a doctor or midwife can try several methods to remove the placenta. The simplest involves pulling very gently on the umbilical cord, which can help some placentas separate. When this doesn't work, the doctor or midwife may need to use a hand slipped into the uterus to help separate a particularly adherent portion of the placenta. Sliding the hand through the cervix into the uterus can be uncomfortable; medication will ease the pain.

Postpartum Bleeding (Bleeding after Delivery)

Every woman has some bleeding for several weeks after a baby is born. On average, about 8 to 10 changes of a menstrual pad are needed during the first 24 hours; within a few days, the number of changes should decrease markedly. When unusually severe bleeding occurs in the first few hours after delivery, the most common reason is that the uterus has not contracted adequately. Contraction of the muscles of the uterus closes off the inside blood vessels, which is how bleeding slows down after delivery. If you have a large amount of bleeding, massaging the lower abdomen will cause the uterus to tighten up. If too much bleeding continues, there are medications that can be given into a vein or by injection to further tighten the uterus.

Increased bleeding more than a day after a baby is born may be caused by infection or by a piece of placenta or membrane that remains in the uterus. An increase in bleeding after childbirth should always be reported promptly to your health-care provider.

21 Relieving the Discomforts of Labor

H aving a baby is not easy. No matter how much it is romanticized in stories, or how significant the event will be for you, there's no avoiding the fact that it is hard work. Labor is intense, and the contractions can be very painful. It often requires you to draw from every energy reserve you have.

Of course, there are women who somehow have a relatively easy time of it (and tell everyone about their experience). These easy labors are partly due to luck, but not entirely. They are most likely to happen to people who are rested, well-informed, in excellent general health, and who have adequate support during labor. As you look ahead to your labor and delivery, we recommend that you not expect a rapid, painless labor. Instead, assume that your labor will be quite intense for many hours. Learn all you can about ways to combat fatigue and pain, and be as well prepared as possible.

You cannot control some factors: the intensity of your contractions, the position of the baby, and the amount of room in your pelvis. All these are important in determining how difficult or easy your labor will be. There is, however, much that you can do to keep from being overwhelmed or overstressed by labor, even if it's long and difficult.

Childbirth Preparation Classes

In 1952, Grantly Dick-Read published *Childbirth Without Fear*, a popular book that launched the natural childbirth movement. In his book, Dr. Dick-Read argued that labor and delivery can be enjoyable and fulfilling. He pointed out that fear and tension, not the contractions themselves, are a major cause of misery during labor (see fig. 44). He also developed a series of classes to inform couples about labor and to teach techniques for alleviating its discomforts. Over the years, his ideas have been expanded and modified by others, including Fernand Lamaze, Robert Bradley, and Sheila Kitzinger.

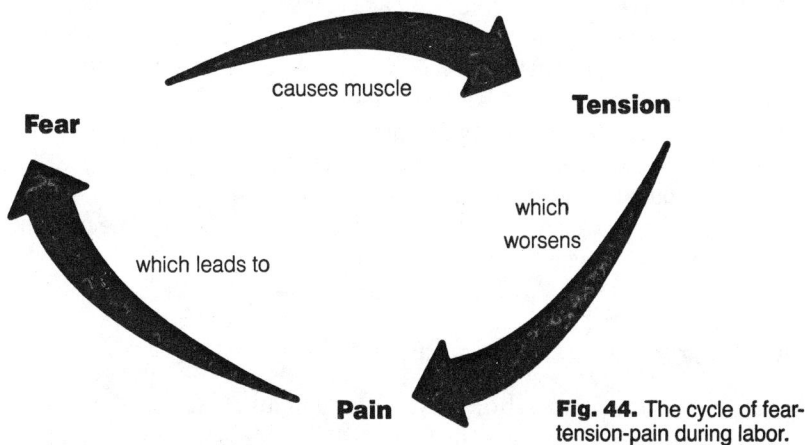

Fear

causes muscle

Tension

which
worsens

which leads to

Pain

Fig. 44. The cycle of fear-tension-pain during labor.

Today, nearly every community has childbirth education classes. Most classes are relatively similar; so, while we encourage you to attend some kind of class, we do not advocate a specific method. If you do have a choice, try to learn about what's available, and then select the class that suits you best.

No matter what kind of class you take, your childbirth education course should inform you about the stages and complications of pregnancy, labor, and delivery, so you will understand what is going on and not be afraid. It should also teach you a specific method of relaxing your body during labor, so you can minimize muscle tension during contractions. All classes teach someone (usually the husband) to be a support person (or coach) for the woman in labor. This support person is vital to the control of pain and discomfort during labor, and he or she should attend every class with the mother-to-be.

In choosing a childbirth preparation class, here are some things to keep in mind:

● If your health-care provider recommends or sponsors a specific class, it is a good idea to take that class. The ideas you learn will then be in tune with your health-care provider's philosophy and practice.

- In general, you will learn more in a class that includes only a few couples than in a large group. A small class provides more individual attention and more opportunity to ask questions.
- All classes teach you to focus your attention during labor on something other than the contractions. Usually, a rhythmic breathing pattern is used to focus attention. This has the added benefit of helping you relax your abdominal, back, leg, and perineal muscles, which lowers your sensation of pain and makes the contractions more effective. The *Lamaze* method teaches several different patterns of breathing that are intended for use during different stages of labor. The *Bradley* method teaches a single type of breathing (deep, slow breathing), which is used throughout labor. Bradley classes begin earlier (in the third month) than most other classes, which usually start in the seventh or eighth month.
- If you have had classes before, you may wish to arrange a brief "refresher" course rather than take a full series of classes.
- Remember to practice your relaxation techniques regularly. The practice will serve you well during labor.

Improving Physical Comfort during Labor

When a woman is in labor, many things can be done to improve her comfort, such as helping her position herself, massaging her back, and applying a warm washcloth to sore muscles. While a support person can provide simple, timely assistance, which will be of great help, the laboring woman can do much to ease her discomfort. Here are some points to keep in mind:

Role of the Support Person (Coach). In the case of all measures meant to relieve the pains of labor, the secret is to use them at the right times. One or more support persons should be constantly attentive during the entire labor. The support person must concentrate on providing comfort in a supportive, but not insistent, way. This requires listening to and being in tune with the woman in labor. Let her be in control, and try to be a perfect servant to her. Let her rest (not talk) between contractions, and help her focus on her breathing and relaxation when she is having a contraction.

Positioning. Finding the most comfortable position at a given moment can make a considerable difference in how a woman copes with labor. Early on, when the contractions are relatively mild, try walking, sitting, rocking, or taking a bath. As contractions intensify, sitting, rocking, or lying down will often be most comfortable. Labor that is most painful in the back (*back labor*) is often relieved by sitting forward, with arms around a support person, or by laboring on hands and knees. Change positions frequently during labor; this improves circulation and helps prevent muscle fatigue.

A Focal Point. Bring something from home to focus on visually during contractions. A sentimental or soothing picture or object is a good choice. It is often helpful to bring a tape player with your favorite music. Many women don't use their focal point, preferring to close their eyes or focus on their coach. But you may get much relief from a focal point; so, choose one to have with you in labor.

Compresses. Early in labor, warm, moist heat feels good on those muscles that are working so hard. Use a washcloth soaked in warm water and place it on the back, neck, or abdomen. Later on, when transition-stage contractions or the efforts at pushing make the laboring woman feel hot, a cool compress will feel soothing on the forehead or abdomen. Change the compresses frequently.

Baths and Showers. If warm compresses provide good relief for aching muscles, a warm bath or shower can feel heavenly. Out of fear of infection, many physicians advise against a tub bath after the membranes have ruptured; but showers are fine at any time.

Massage. Deep muscle massage is often very effective in labor. It is especially helpful for back labor and for helping muscles relax at the end of a contraction. Since it is only helpful when it feels good, the woman and her support person need to communicate about what feels good and what doesn't. Some women in labor do not like to be touched at all, even though they still need emotional support; most women don't like to be touched much during transition.

A coach massaging a woman in labor should use baby powder, talc, or corn starch to help the hands slide more smoothly. We recommend powders because oils and lotions build up into a gooey mess if used for several hours. The exception is when the baby's head has moved down so far that it stretches the labia (a situation called crowning). At that time, it is helpful to massage the perineum with a small amount of mineral or baby oil.

Often, women feel labor pains with particular intensity in the lower back (like a *very* severe menstrual cramp). When this occurs, strong, steady pressure often feels best, applied with the thumbs or the heel of the hand in the areas marked in figure 45. Don't be surprised if the best spot shifts somewhat from one contraction to the next.

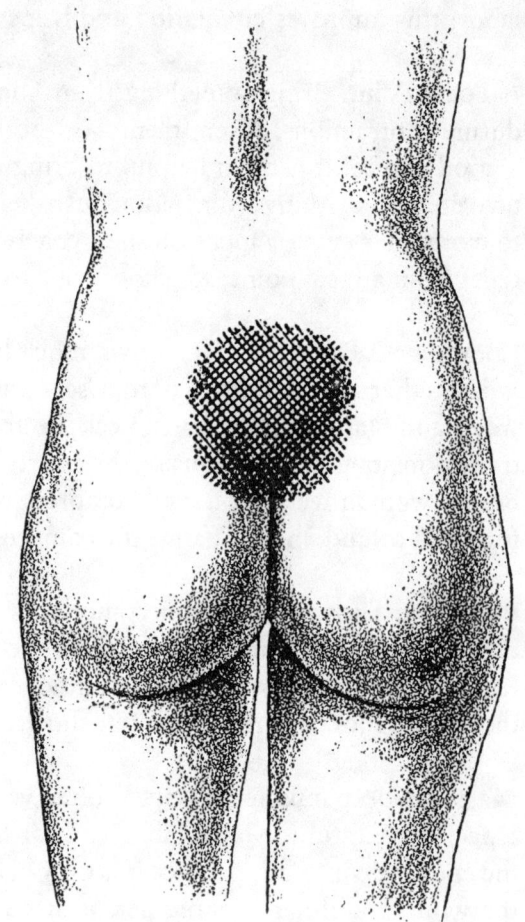

Fig. 45. Where to apply pressure to relieve back pressure.

Effleurage. Many women in labor get a lot of relief from very light brushing of the abdomen during a contraction. This form of massage, called effleurage (a French term meaning "feather touch"), can be done by the woman in labor or by the support person. Use one or two hands, and ever so lightly brush the surface of the abdomen with your fingertips. Move in a circle around the belly button.

Resting between Contractions. Labor can be so intense, with such concentration needed during contractions, that a woman can tire quickly. It is important to rest between contractions. As a contraction fades, there will often be some leftover muscle tension. Wring it out of your body by consciously taking a long, deep breath, and relaxing every muscle of the body as the breath is slowly let out.

This long, relaxing breath (often called a "cleansing breath") should end each contraction. It should be followed by a time of relaxing, often with eyes closed, to gather energy for the next contraction.

Keeping the Mouth Moist. As labor moves on, dryness of the mouth and lips can result from breathing heavily during contractions. Ice chips or slushy drinks to cool and moisten should be available and offered frequently. Lollipops are helpful too; they moisten the mouth and provide a little sugar for energy. They are better than hard candies, because a lollipop can be taken out of the mouth easily when a contraction begins.

Packing a Labor Bag. As the due date approaches, you should gather together the items you may use to provide comfort during labor. For a list of items, see the checklist on page 261. As a reference about labor, take along the Notes for the Coach on pages 262–63.

A Supportive Atmosphere for the Woman in Labor

Labor goes best when the woman can concentrate and is given good support. For this reason, it is important to create and maintain an atmosphere of caring.

The room itself should be relaxed, homelike, and quiet. Low lighting is often helpful, and music from home can add a relaxing touch. Privacy should be preserved as much as possible. The bed should be comfortable, and there should be places for the coach, other support persons, and the woman in labor to sit.

Tips for Coaches

Everyone who helps the woman in labor should try to be in tune with her experience, to anticipate her needs, and to provide for them. Remember that talking takes energy and concentration, so don't try to carry on a conversation during strong labor or ask questions during a contraction. Encourage her to rely on her instincts and feelings, and to communicate them to others. When the contractions are intense, remind her to focus on each one individually, then relax and gather her strength.

Much of the time, the coach does not need to do anything physical to aid or comfort the laboring woman. He (or she) should always be there, however, reminding her to relax, helping her breathe, and letting her feel free to ask for anything that will make her more comfortable. Whenever the coach must leave her side, someone else should fill in.

When coaching a woman in labor, use simple, direct instructions. Remind her how far her labor has progressed and what to expect next. Tell her exactly what to do, so she can do it without having to think. For example, if she is pushing before it's time, tell her to "pant" or "blow out," rather than to "stop pushing." When she is contracting, don't talk to anyone else. Help her pace her breathing by looking at her and breathing with her, if she finds this helpful. Encourage her with statements like "it's halfway over," "you can do it," or "good." When the contraction is over, remind her to take a deep, cleansing breath. Help her relax with statements like "let your body go limp and relaxed," or "pretend that you are sleeping in the sun, and rest . . . I love you."

If you are the coach, you should be on the lookout for two signs of particular discomfort:

● Tightness of any of her muscles during or after a contraction. When you see this, gently remind her to relax.
● A look of distress (however fleeting). When you see this, ask her what is bothering her (you may need to wait until the contraction is over). Then try to help her resolve it. If you cannot help her, talk to the nurse or to your health-care provider. Resolving her pain or concern will help labor go better.

Medications

There are various medications that can be used to provide pain relief in labor. As you plan your labor, speak with your health-care provider about the medications he or she commonly uses.

Narcotics. Narcotics, such as Demerol, are strong pain relievers that can be given as an injection, usually through an intravenous (i.v.) line. They work quickly (within about 15 minutes) and can be given as frequently as necessary to control pain. Narcotics do not entirely take away the discomfort of contractions, but they make it less intense. In addition, they may make you drowsy. This helps provide relaxation between contractions, but it can cause you to be slow to start your breathing when a new contraction comes (the coach will need to remind you to do so). Narcotics make it more difficult to push, and can cause newborns to be sluggish at taking their first breaths. For these reasons, they should be timed to wear off (they last between two and four hours) by the second stage of labor. If necessary, the effect of a narcotic can be rapidly reversed by giving a second medication (Narcan).

Medications for Nausea. Medications such as Phenargen are generally given with a narcotic, because they help make it more effective and combat a major side effect of narcotics, nausea.

Spinal. A "spinal" involves giving a medication like novocaine through a needle into the back. The medication numbs all the nerves in the lower abdomen and the perineum. Because it produces such intense numbness, it generally makes pushing very difficult. Its use is now relatively limited, because it is less safe than narcotics or epidural anesthesia, but it can be used to provide excellent pain relief during a forceps delivery.

Epidural. An epidural is a variation of the spinal in which a thin plastic tube is threaded through a needle into the space just outside the spinal nerves. This allows medication to be given every few hours to numb the lower abdomen and perineum. It is safer than a spinal, but it must be administered by an anesthesiologist. It is particularly useful for women who have unusually painful contractions from early on in labor, because it can provide excellent relief for a long period of time. Pushing is somewhat more difficult, but an epidural can be timed to wear off so you can push. Side effects include lowering of the blood pressure, numbness of the legs, and (if the spinal canal is accidently entered) headache.

Inhalation Methods. In the past, women in labor were commonly put to sleep during labor. This is rarely done any more, because complications are much more frequent. When general anesthetics are used, a forceps delivery is more often necessary, reactions to medication can occur, and the baby may have breathing problems. Thus, although an intense labor may make you wish you could just be put to sleep, this is generally not advised for medical reasons. There are some situations, however, in which certain mild gases (such as nitrous oxide) are used during labor. Even these, which do not put you to sleep, make it impossible to concentrate enough to use any of the more basic methods of pain relief, such as relaxing, focusing, and breathing.

Pudental Block. This is a method of numbing the perineum during the last few minutes of pushing, as the head is crowning. It involves injecting a numbing medication (such as Xylocaine) into an area deep in your vagina, where the nerves from the perineum are close to the surface.

When used properly, medication can help you rest during labor. This will make it easier for you to be alert and awake when it's time to push. Since the goal of care during labor should be the birth of a healthy baby to a healthy mother, you should not consider appropriate use of medication as an experience inferior to natural childbirth. If your labor requires this help, be glad it is available.

On the other hand, do seek to use medication only if it's really needed. Natural methods can preserve your energy with far fewer risks and side effects. They work well for most people, put you and your partner more in control of labor, and will allow you to regain your strength quickly after delivery.

RECOMMENDED RESOURCES

Dick-Read, Grantly. *Childbirth Without Fear.* 4th Edition. New York: Harper & Row, 1972. The classic book that popularized natural methods of childbirth.

Ewy, Donna and Roger. *Preparation for Childbirth.* 3d Edition. New York: Signet Books, 1982. A small, readable, and practical introduction to Lamaze techniques.

Walker, Morton, Bernice Yoffe, and Parke Gray. *The Complete Book of Birth.* New York: Simon and Schuster, 1979. A detailed discussion of the various childbirth preparation methods.

22 Helping to Plan Your Childbirth

P arents today tend to regard childbirth as a natural process, while recognizing that specialized medical treatment may need to be a part of the process. They learn, from reading and talking to friends, that health-care providers often disagree on how much technology to use in the care of normal labor and delivery. Frequently, parents-to-be hear or read about childbirth experiences in which a couple was unhappy with the kind of care they received.

As you learn about the childbirth process, you will develop your own views about how you would like things to go. To avoid the kind of disappointment you may have heard about, we recommend that you and your health-care provider begin to build an understanding at the time you first meet.

The best way to plan the childbirth experience you want is to talk it over with your health-care provider. Find out what routines are used in his or her practice, what policies the hospital has, and what choices are available to you. Let your health-care provider know your feelings and preferences. Whether you go to an obstetrician, a family physician, or a midwife, your health-care provider should be accustomed to answering questions about labor and delivery from concerned parents-to-be. By discussing these issues during prenatal care, you will come to a better understanding, and the stage will be set for open communication when decisions must be made during labor.

Not all parents-to-be want to plan the details of their childbirth; many prefer to leave this up to the health-care provider. Others are interested in general philosophy but not in specific details. We rec-

ommend that you read the following list of questions carefully to
become familiar with the kinds of choices that can be made. Then
decide to what extent you wish to discuss these with your health-
care provider.

Twenty-one Questions about Labor and Delivery

**1. What admission routines does the hospital have? Does the
staff routinely give enemas or shave the pubic area?**

2. Is there a choice of labor rooms in the hospital?
Many hospitals allow you to choose between "home-style" rooms and the
more traditional labor rooms.

**3. How many people—and which ones—may be with me
during labor?**
All hospitals have rules about the number of people who are permitted to
be in the room with a woman in labor. Some require classes for all individuals
who plan to be present.

**4. What are the rules about children being present during
labor and delivery? Are there any facilities available for
children?**

5. To what extent can I eat and drink during labor?
Food in the stomach tends not to be digested in labor. In addition, nausea
and vomiting are common during labor. For these reasons, all health-care
providers limit what you can take in during labor. There are, however,
differences in the extent of these restrictions, depending on the health-care
provider.

**6. Do you routinely give intravenous (i.v.) fluids to women in
labor? If not, what are the situations in which you decide to use
an i.v.?**

**7. How commonly do you use electronic monitoring for
women in labor?**

8. What are your approaches to pain relief during labor?
It is quite common for women to underestimate how much discomfort they
will have, particularly with their first labor, which tends to be the most difficult.
The best way of preparing for this aspect of labor, in addition to exercising
and learning a method such as Lamaze, is to discuss and understand your
pain-relief options beforehand. Review our discussion of pain relief during
labor (chapter 21); then go over the details with your health-care provider.

**9. To what extent will you talk things over with me before
choosing pain medication during my labor?**

**10. If my contractions are not strong enough, do you try
nipple stimulation before using a medication such as oxytocin?**
Nipple stimulation releases natural oxytocin, the same chemical that is
given intravenously to stimulate labor. It is performed by having the woman or

her partner gently roll the nipple between two fingers. It has been used for centuries and often seems to be effective in stimulating labor.

11. What can I bring from home to make labor more comfortable?

Examples include pillows, lollipops, and a tape player with your favorite music. Your childbirth instructor may have more to say about this than your physician or midwife.

12. How do you routinely position the mother during delivery? Will you offer me a choice?

In this country, delivery with the mother on her back was just about the only position used for many years. But a variety of positions are suitable. Common alternative positions include lying on the left side, squatting with some kind of support such as a birthing chair, and semi-squatting (propped up, usually with pillows).

13. Can the lights be dimmed during delivery of the baby and for a few minutes afterwards?

The theory behind this practice is that babies' eyes are quite sensitive to light after being in the darkness of the womb, and that a dimly lit delivery room would be preferred by the newborn.

14. Do you provide Leboyer-style delivery?

Dr. Frederick Leboyer is a French obstetrician who developed and popularized a childbirth method involving delivery in a dim room and placing the child in a warm bath soon after birth.

15. Under what circumstances do you perform an episiotomy during delivery?

The episiotomy is a cut made with surgical scissors to enlarge the opening of the vagina and let the baby come out more easily. It is currently the object of much debate.

Many physicians feel that episiotomy shortens the last phase of labor, prevents serious lacerations, and may decrease the potential for birth injury to the baby when performed on women who presumably need it. Some also believe that episiotomy helps prevent bladder problems in later years by reducing injury to the muscles and nerves that support the bladder.

Other physicians, and most midwives, feel that episiotomies are generally not necessary. They find that many women can deliver without an episiotomy, and that lacerations, when they develop, heal quickly and with less pain than the average episiotomy. Health-care providers with this approach are likely to prefer a slower delivery with stretching of the perineum and the potential for spontaneous rather than artificial cutting of the perineum.

16. After the baby is born, do you clamp the umbilical cord immediately or wait before doing so?

There is no consistent opinion about what is best. Waiting a minute or two before clamping the cord usually allows extra blood to flow from the placenta to the baby. The debate is over whether this extra blood is good, bad, or of no consequence, because both too little and too much blood can cause complications. If you have a strong preference about this, we recommend discussing it with your health-care provider.

17. Can I hold my baby and attempt to breastfeed right after delivery?

Many babies are not hungry right after being born, but the contact is always good.

18. How soon after delivery will my baby be taken to the nursery? For how long will he or she have to stay there?

Nursery staff do many important things such as weighing, examining, and giving vitamin K to newborns. Often there can be flexibility in their routines. If desired, the performance of routine nursery activities can be delayed for a time after birth. In addition, some childbirth settings allow all or some of these routines to be done right in the delivery room.

19. Can my baby have antibiotic drops other than silver nitrate put in his or her eyes?

By law, antibiotic drops must be placed in the eyes of all newborns to prevent gonorrhea eye infection, which can cause blindness. Silver nitrate has been traditionally used, but it often causes the eyes to be red, swollen, and sensitive to light for a couple of days. Tetracycline or erythromycin can be used instead, and both are milder.

20. Is rooming-in available?

Rooming-in is an option available in many hospitals that allows a baby to be with its mother all or most of the time.

21. If I need a caesarean section, will I have a choice of being put to sleep versus having a spinal? What are your opinions about anesthesia during caesarean section? Will my partner be allowed to stay with me while the operation is performed?

Few people plan to deliver by caesarean section, but between 10 and 15 percent of deliveries occur this way. The movement to make childbirth a more natural process has extended to caesarean birth, too. Often, you can be awake during the delivery, with your partner present, and you can hold your baby minutes after delivery. As you discuss your upcoming delivery with your health-care provider, the possibility of caesarean birth should not be omitted.

RECOMMENDED READING

Leboyer, Frederick. *Childbirth Without Violence*. New York: Alfred A. Knopf, 1975. A classic book, written by the obstetrician who developed the technique of delivery using dim lighting and placing the newborn in a warm bath.

Simkin, Penny, Jane Whalley, and Ann Keppler. *Pregnancy, Childbirth and the Newborn*. Deep Haven, Minnesota: Meadowbrook Books, 1984. The first chapter of this book is devoted to negotiating your childbirth with your health-care provider.

PART V

You and Your New Baby

23 The New Mother's Hospital Experience

Your baby has been born and you are now resting comfortably in your room. It is hard to imagine what has just happened, and no one else can describe the experience you have just had. Those first moments with your child in your arms are an occasion you will never forget. Most of the time the feelings of wonder and love will ease the pain or memory of difficulties during labor. If you do not remember the details of your labor and delivery, don't be embarrassed to ask your delivery nurse, physician, midwife, partner, or support person. Knowing the story of your delivery and who was involved with your care will help you in the future to plan or to cope with other medical situations that might arise.

Birth Certificates, Names, and Other Hospital Paperwork

Shortly after delivery, baby and mother will be given duplicate name bands to wear on their arms. These bands with identification numbers serve as legal proof of parenthood to avoid any confusion. Upon discharge from the hospital, you will have to sign a form that verifies that the child you are taking home is your own. Although it may seem silly to worry about such things, checking the numbers on the name band is a good idea.

In most states, births are recorded formally on a state certificate. Typically, a birth certificate has the mother's maiden name, married name, the father's name, the parents' address, their ages and race, and information about the baby's condition at the time of birth. If the mother and father are not legally married, the father's name can still be entered on the birth certificate.

Within the first 24 hours of your delivery, a birth recorder will visit you to obtain the data that will appear on the birth certificate. At this time you may give the name of your child if you have chosen one, but you don't have to name your child immediately after delivery. Depending on the state in which you live, you have between seven days and several years to record the name of your child on the official birth certificate. If you do choose a name and have it entered on the birth certificate and then decide to change it, you can do so by filing a name change with the state recorder of vital statistics. The birth certificate you sign in the hospital will be sent to the state office of vital statistics to be officially recorded. You will be given a form to send in to this office requesting an official copy of the birth certificate for your own records. In most states, this service is free. However, if there is a name change, there may be a fee involved. Check with your birth recorder after delivery for specifics.

Other papers you will be given to sign or read may include consent forms for rubella immunization (if the mother was not already immunized prior to pregnancy), consent forms for RhoGAM injections (if the mother is Rh-negative and the baby is Rh-positive), consent forms for circumcision, and information sheets on postpartum exercises, hygiene, episiotomy care, and family planning. It may seem like a lot of paper, but it is well worth saving these items and reading them when you have a spare minute.

Bonding

Bonding is the term used to describe the attachment that develops between the parents and baby when they are together in the hours and days after birth. While this term is often applied to the time just after delivery, bonding develops between parents and newborn over days and months. The birth of a baby signifies, in fact, the birth of a family or a significant family change. When a child is born, each family member needs to bond with the new individual. Relationships in the family change to adjust to the new member. These changes are usually healthy ones and reflect the maturing of the family itself. As parents, you will see changes in your relationship, as well as in your feelings about yourselves as individuals.

Bonding has a positive ring to it, and the trend in most health-care institutions is to help develop a positive relationship between the new parents and their baby. Techniques sometimes used to enhance bonding include placing the baby on the mother's abdomen immediately after delivery, having the father clamp and cut the cord, having the father bathe the baby after delivery, and placing an infant delivered by caeserean section in its mother's arms. Bonding is enhanced by later contact as well, such as when the new baby takes the breast for the first time, when the father accomplishes his first diaper change, or during those special first moments at home.

As parents and baby bond and get to know each other, the parents begin to assume their roles as mother and father. If they are first-time parents, this can mean a significant change in role for each. If one parent (or both) is having difficulty in dealing with these changes, then the quality of bonding can be affected. Often an outside person can observe problems that you may not be able to see; a good friend, relative, physician, midwife, or nurse may comment and offer suggestions. If you feel that you need help in thinking about issues now that the baby is here, or if you are just worried about how things seem to be going, feel free to ask others you trust for help.

Premature Babies

If your baby was one of the 7 or 8 percent born before 37 weeks, he or she may need extra hospital care. The type of care depends on the baby's weight and physical maturity. In general, babies born after 34 weeks do very well, babies born before 28 weeks do poorly, and babies born during the weeks between require varying amounts of nursing and mechanical life-support to grow.

If your baby was born prematurely, your experience in the hospital may be different than with the delivery of a full-term baby. For example, immediately after delivery, you may not be able to hold your newborn because a pediatrician needs to examine the premature infant. In most hospitals, parents have access to their children 24 hours a day, even if they are in a neonatal intensive care nursery. Children born five or six weeks early are often put in intensive care units for close observation since they are prone to having problems with feeding, temperature maintenance, and breathing.

On page 264, you will find delivery and birth information charts on which you can record for yourself the basic details of your childbirth.

Hospital Care for the Mother

Some mothers feel exhilirated and energetic after delivery, whereas others feel quite tired. The time immediately after delivery is a special time for the new parents to become adjusted to their baby and to relax before a busy period of speaking to relatives and running errands. Many couples need this privacy. We suggest that you use the time in the hospital to rest and to get ready to meet the outside world.

Immediately after your delivery, a nurse will help you into a clean hospital gown, or onto clean sheets and back into a comfortable position. Every 10 to 15 minutes, she will check your blood pressure, note the amount of bleeding, and massage your uterus to prevent excessive bleeding. Most of the control of bleeding after delivery is accomplished by the uterus, a remarkable muscle that contracts very quickly after delivery. If you have an intravenous line (i.v.), you will probably receive oxytocin, a hormone that speeds uterine contraction. If bleeding is prolonged after delivery, another drug called Methergine may be given; it causes rather intense uterine contractions.

Most women feel small contractions through the first few days after delivery. You may feel these "afterpains" more intensely when breastfeeding because nursing releases oxytocin. Sometimes, afterpains are severe enough to require medication for relief. If you have painful contractions after delivery, do not be afraid to ask your nurse for medication.

If you had an episiotomy, the nurse will place some ice between your vulvar area and the sanitary pad. Although it feels cold, the ice pack decreases the amount of labial swelling and relieves pain in this area. Later on, exposing the episiotomy site to a warm heat lamp will speed healing. Ask your nurse to bring you one if you are uncomfortable. The heat is quite healing to the area and brings immediate relief. Don't be afraid to get up even if your episiotomy hurts; you'll heal faster if you move about.

After delivery some women find that they have trouble emptying their bladders. This is usually due to swelling of the labia around the urethra or bruising of the urethra during the delivery. If you are having a lot of difficulty and pain with urination, you may be asked to sit in a sitz bath and try to urinate into the water. If you simply cannot empty your bladder, tell the nurse. It may be necessary to have a small rubber or plastic tube called a catheter placed into the bladder to empty it. When the catheter is placed in the urethra, you may feel a sharp pain for two to three seconds, much like the pain one experiences with severe bladder infections. It takes about 90 seconds to empty the bladder and to have the catheter removed. Once the bladder is emptied in this manner, you should have no more difficulty passing urine. In a few instances, this catheterization may need to be repeated, or the catheter may need to remain within the bladder for a day or two until the swelling subsides. Trouble passing urine is slightly more common among women who have epidural anesthesia, because the nerves that control urination have been anesthetized also. This problem diminishes as the epidural anesthetic wears off.

Most physicians and midwives encourage their patients to breast-feed and will suggest putting the baby to breast soon after birth. Most nurseries will cooperate by getting the baby back to the mother as soon as possible after delivery. Although your milk will not come in for two or three days after delivery, the breasts secrete at the time of birth colostrum, a watery liquid containing protein and antibodies. Most healthy babies can suck well enough to benefit from this protein-rich substance. The more sucking the baby does, the sooner milk is produced and breastfeeding can begin in earnest.

Many hospitals allow a healthy baby to "room in," which means that a baby remains with the mother during the stay in the hospital. Some hospitals do not permit this until 24 hours after delivery, so that nurses and doctors in the nursery can observe the newborn closely. Other hospitals permit rooming-in to begin immediately after a child has been examined by a physician. With premature babies, who require closer observation of their temperature and breathing cycles, rooming-in is usually not an option.

Rooming-in gives the mother and father the responsibility for looking after a new baby with the nursery personnel available to assist as needed. Rooming-in is offered to parents as long as the baby is doing well. If a baby is rooming in, the only visitors permitted into the room are the father and grandparents; other visitors can view the baby through the nursery window. There are pros and cons to rooming-in and the choice is not irrevocable. Some hospitals offer a combination of the two: rooming-in during the day, and staying in the nursery at night. This provides the mother with an opportunity to get some much needed uninterrupted sleep if she so desires.

As part of the hospital routine, nurses will check the postpartum mother's temperature and blood pressure every four to six hours.

They will also ask about bleeding, constipation, and problems with urination. The mother's blood count will probably be checked once after delivery, or more often if there was significant blood loss. Also, the pediatric nurses will look in to see how mother and baby are doing at breastfeeding, diaper changes, care of the umbilical cord, and other activities. These nurses can provide valuable information and guidance, so feel free to ask your nurse for help.

Your physician or midwife will visit you at least once a day to examine you and to answer questions. He or she will check your breasts for engorgement, milk production, and infection, note the size of your uterus, examine the perineum for swelling, check the episiotomy or laceration repair (if it was done during delivery), and inquire about excessive bleeding. If you have other complaints or problems, be sure to ask your health-care provider at this time.

How long you stay in the hospital depends on the condition of you and your baby, the hospital rules, the philosophy of the health-care provider, and the wishes of the parents. Some hospitals prefer 24 hours of observation for new babies, but if your health-care provider will see the baby at daily intervals, there usually is no problem with early discharge. Experienced parents may feel comfortable with discharge before 24 hours; however, new parents may want to use the two- or three-day stay in the hospital as a time to gain confidence in taking care of the new infant.

Normal Body Changes after Delivery

Although your body changes a lot in a very short time after delivery, many women feel upset that they do not immediately look the way they did before becoming pregnant. Remember that it took nine months for your body to accommodate to the presence of a full-term baby; it will take some time, usually a few months, for you to regain your shape and to feel as you did before you became pregnant.

After delivery, you may be concerned that you still look pregnant. This is common, because the uterus stays enlarged for several weeks after delivery (see fig. 46). In addition, the stomach muscles and skin have been stretched along with the pelvic muscles, and they need time to regain their tone. You can begin exercises a week or so after delivery to tone up these muscles. Also, breastfeeding will keep the uterus well contracted and speed its return to normal size.

You urinate quite frequently in the first day or two after delivery

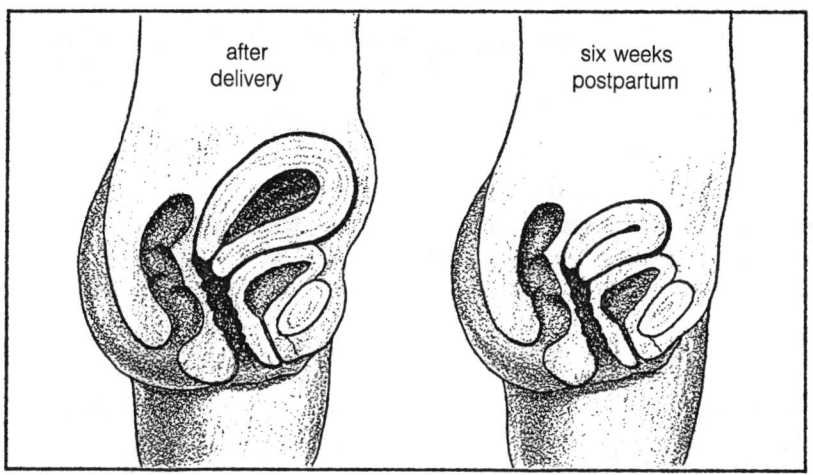

Fig. 46. Normal body changes. Immediately after delivery the uterus is still enlarged; it shrinks or "involutes" over the next six weeks.

as your body gets rid of the extra fluid it has stored during these last nine months. You may also notice increased perspiration and thirst as the body works hard to produce milk. Many women find that they need to drink a lot more fluid while they are breastfeeding to compensate for the milk they are producing.

The breasts become fuller, warmer, heavier, and more tender as they fill with milk in preparation for breastfeeding and in response to the new baby's sucking (see fig. 47). The heaviness and warmth of the breasts usually resolves after a regular schedule of breastfeeding is established.

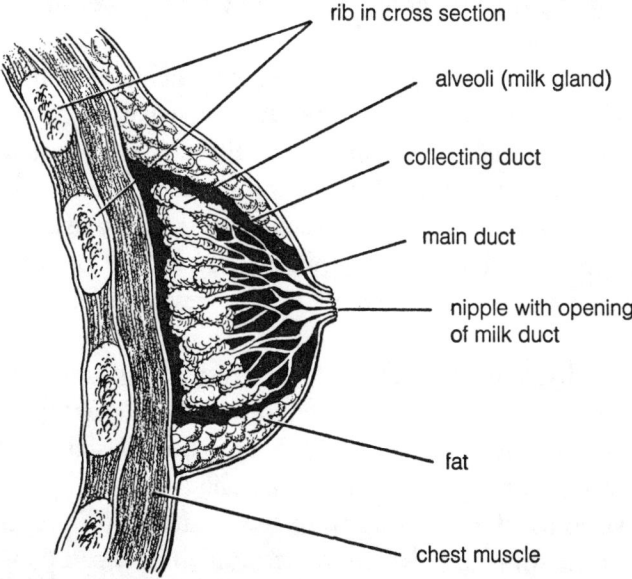

Fig. 47. Lactating breast. As the baby sucks, milk is drawn into collecting ducts, through the main ducts, and out through the nipple

179

Giving birth, caring full-time for a new baby, and experiencing major changes in your body can leave you exhausted. The body's requirements for emotional and physical rest, water, and food are different. Also, changes in the levels of certain hormones (particularly estrogen and progesterone) cause some women to feel depressed, which is often called postpartum blues. This very real phenomenon—postpartum depression, or baby blues—will be discussed in a separate section (see page 226).

Feeling Dehumanized or Uncomfortable

Most people who enter a hospital for any kind of treatment feel as if they are giving up control of their lives. Nurses and doctors tell you what to do and what to eat, as well as when you can get out of bed, use the bathroom, move around the room, or even sit up. The smallest thing you are used to doing for yourself may not be permissible or possible when you enter the hospital as a patient. Even though giving birth is not an illness, it is considered a "procedure," and like every procedure that is performed in a hospital, there are rules and regulations that apply to it. Feeling dehumanized is common for most patients, but especially for new mothers who consider giving birth an activity over which *they* should have control. These feelings can be minimized by discussing beforehand with your health-care provider the rules and regulations surrounding delivery in your hospital or birth center. If you anticipate communication problems, ask a friend or family member to help you voice your feelings either before you enter the birthing facility or during your stay in the facility.

There is also a loss of privacy that occurs around delivery. While many women in labor do not notice the frequent presence of strangers in the labor room or delivery room, after delivery most women notice the lack of privacy and feel a bit uncomfortable about it. If you are a patient in a teaching hospital, remember that you usually may specify by whom you wish to be treated. You have a right to request that treatment only be given by your own health-care providers.

Other physical discomforts, such as pain from episiotomy repair, from uterine contractions, or from engorged breasts, are normal but may be quite severe. After most deliveries the physician or midwife will arrange for a pain medication to be available by request—you have to ask for medication to receive it. If you are in pain and there is not an order already written, any nurse can contact your health-care provider to obtain one for you. There are safe medications for pain that you can take while breastfeeding. There are also many remedies that do not involve drugs, such as sitz baths, breastbinders and ice packs for nonbreastfeeding mothers, and warm compresses for breastfeeding mothers. All you need to do is ask.

RECOMMENDED RESOURCES

Anderson, Mary. *Pregnancy after Thirty*. London: Faber and Faber, 1984. A good resource for older mothers. Short and easy to read.

Boston Women's Health Book Collective. *Our Bodies, Ourselves: A Book by and for Women*. New York: Simon and Schuster, 1976. A book to read over and over again, with an excellent overview of pregnancy and delivery. Personal vignettes and poetry are interspersed with a tremendous amount of helpful information.

Whelan, Elizabeth. *Pregnancy Survival Guide*. Wasuwatosa, Wis.: American Baby Books, 1978. A must for a new mother. A practical book that gives you an overview of pregnancy and delivery. This book has many helpful suggestions.

24 The Baby in the Hospital

A newborn baby needs to do many things that it did not have to do while in the womb. These new activities include maintaining temperature, breathing, and eating. Immediately after birth, the birth attendant will check the ability of the baby to sustain itself. If the baby is having trouble breathing, the baby's mouth will be suctioned out and oxygen will be offered, if needed. A heated incubator or a blanket will be used to keep the baby warm.

Attendants will grade the condition of the baby at one minute and five minutes of age using the Apgar Scale (fig. 48). This 10-point rating scale, named for Virginia Apgar, the physician who developed it, provides a way to assess the baby's condition right after birth. The rating indicates how well the baby tolerated labor and whether special medical attention is needed.

If all is well with the new baby, he or she will be left with you for a while. Footprints and identification bands will be made; you'll get a band that matches the baby's. At some point, the baby will be taken to the nursery for weighing and bathing. In the nursery, either silver nitrate drops or other antibiotic drops or ointment will be placed in the eyes to prevent infection. Most hospitals give the baby an injection of vitamin K to help in blood clotting. The baby's blood may also be measured for glucose content and hematocrit. The baby's temperature, respiratory rate, heart rate, and characteristics of breathing must be observed every three to four hours. In addition, the nursery staff will note the newborn's sucking ability and feeding and elimination (urine and stool) patterns. If all is well, the baby can remain with its parents, depending on the hospital's rooming-in policy and the mother's ability to provide care.

Somewhere between the second and fourth days of life, blood will be taken to screen for certain hereditary diseases that can cause mental retardation. This single test, done by taking blood via a heel stick, looks for several diseases. The PKU test measures phenylalanine levels in the baby's blood. If these levels are exceptionally high, the baby can be placed on a special diet to prevent retardation. Other substances tested for in the blood include galactose, thyroid hormone, homocystine, histidine, and tyrosine. Each of these is a marker for a specific disease that can cause mental retardation. All can be corrected with treatment.

Apgar Scale

Item Tested	0	1 point	2 points
Heart Rate	absent	slow (less than 100 beats per minute)	100 beats or more per minute
Breathing	absent	slow or irregular	regular
Muscle Tone	limp	some motion of extremities	active motion
Skin Color	blue, pale	pink body blue extremities	pink all over
Reflex Response	no response	grimace	vigorous cry

Fig. 48. The Apgar Scale. This standard measurement of a baby's condition immediately after birth is taken at one and five minutes after delivery. Scores of 7–10 indicate that the baby is healthy. Scores of 4–7 indicate a need for medical intervention. Scores of 0–4 indicate a need for resuscitation and artificial ventilation.

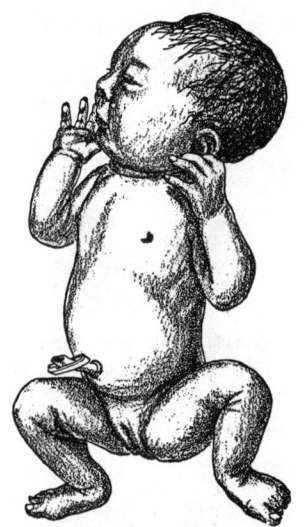

How Does a New Baby Look?

When you first see your new baby, he or she will not look like the picture of the babies on the cover of child-care books or on the labels of baby food jars (see fig. 49). He or she may be covered with blood and amniotic fluid, and in some cases with vernix, a cheese-like substance that protects the baby's skin while inside the uterus. The newborn's skin may be covered by fine dark hair, called lanugo, which will disappear in the first two months of life. The skin color may initially seem dark blue but as the baby begins to breathe it should change to a healthy pink. Most babies cry at birth, al-

Fig. 49. How a newborn looks immediately after birth.

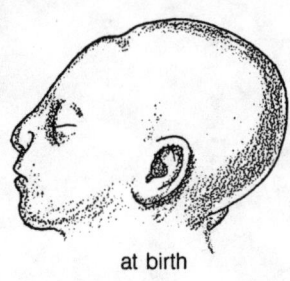

at birth

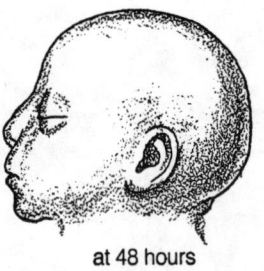

at 48 hours

Fig. 50. The shape of a newborn's head at birth and at 48 hours after birth.

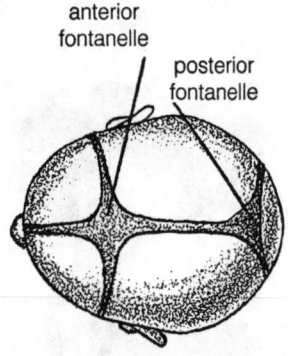

anterior
fontanelle

posterior
fontanelle

Fig. 51. Fontanelles, the intersections of the bones of the skull.

though some begin to breathe very quietly. When a baby doesn't take a breath immediately, the birth attendant may rub its back or massage its heels to stimulate breathing.

The head of the newborn often looks misshapen and pointed as a result of the journey through the birth canal. This temporary shaping of the head, called molding, is possible because the baby has five head bones held together by tough membranes (fig. 50). This arrangement is flexible, allowing the head to change shape to better fit through the mother's pelvis. If the second stage of labor was prolonged, you may notice a lump on the baby's head, called a caput, formed when the baby's head pushed through the dilated cervix. This lump will disappear in the first 48 hours of life.

The new infant's head will seem large in comparison with its body. In fact, the head is usually as big around as the chest at birth. On top of the head is a spot called the anterior fontanelle, where the edges of four bones come together but don't quite meet. There is also another fontanelle at the back of the head, the posterior fontanelle, which is much smaller. Both are covered by a thick membrane and are very sturdy (fig. 51). As the baby grows, these spots get smaller and eventually disappear. The posterior fontanelle closes a few months after birth, and the anterior fontanelle disappears by 18 months.

The face of a newborn often looks flattened, with the ears, nose, and cheeks appearing creased or bruised. These creases and bruises usually fade within the first day of life as the baby recovers from delivery. Many babies are born with a full head of hair. Often this hair falls out during the first few months of life, to grow back (sometimes lighter in color) later. The neck of the newborn may appear quite short and hidden. The umbilical cord, which brought blood to and from the placenta, becomes translucent and feels gelatinous after being cut. As the stump of the cord dries, it becomes yellow, and eventually falls off.

Many boy and girl babies have small breasts that occasionally produce a milky discharge. This is a result of the high level of estrogen in placental blood during pregnancy. For the same reason, the genitals of the newborn often appear swollen, and some girl babies have a small amount of vaginal bleeding during the first few days of life. The breast swelling, as well as the milky discharge (if there has been any), will disappear in the first few weeks of life. The breasts should be left alone to prevent infection.

If the baby is full-term, its fingernails will be fully developed. If the baby arrives late, the nails may be very long. Newborns with long nails often scratch their faces; so you may well wish to trim the nails within the first few days. Cut them with small scissors, file them with an emery board, or carefully bite them. Often the nursery will place mittens on a newborn's hands to prevent the nails from scratching the face.

At delivery, the hands and feet will be darker than the other parts of the body, but they will become pinker as the baby gets older. You will notice creases and lines along the skin folds. Legs and arms are usually flexed as a result of being curled up inside the mother; they remain so for the first few months.

A Newborn's Reflexes

Newborns have several reflexes at birth (fig. 52), which physicians often check, because their presence shows that the baby's central nervous system is intact. Touching the baby's lips produces the *sucking reflex*. If one stimulates the roof of the baby's mouth, the suck will become even stronger. (Physicians and mothers often use this maneuver to quiet the new baby when it cries.) The *rooting reflex* is tested by gently touching the baby's cheek: the baby turns its head toward the side that was stimulated, and the lips move toward the stimulus and attempt to suck it. This reflex facilitates breastfeeding. The *grasp reflex* is produced by touching the baby's palm. The baby's finger will then curl around whatever is touching the palm; pulling against the grip will strengthen the baby's grasp. There is a modified grasp reflex in the feet, which can be produced by stroking the sole of the foot. The toes will then curl around the stimulus.

Though an infant cannot stand alone until about one year of age, there is a *walking reflex* that can be produced by holding the baby upright and having the feet contact a firm surface. The baby will then appear to be walking, although with rather uncoordinated movements. The most commonly observed reflex is the *Moro reflex*, or *startle reflex*: when jostled or upon hearing a loud noise, the baby throws out both arms and spreads its hands widely.

All of these reflexes test the baby's nervous system and its functioning. The walking reflex tests the ability of the newborn to move its legs, the Moro tests the arm movements, the suck and root test whether the baby is able to feed appropriately. As the baby grows and its nervous system develops more fully, these and other "primitive reflexes" will disappear.

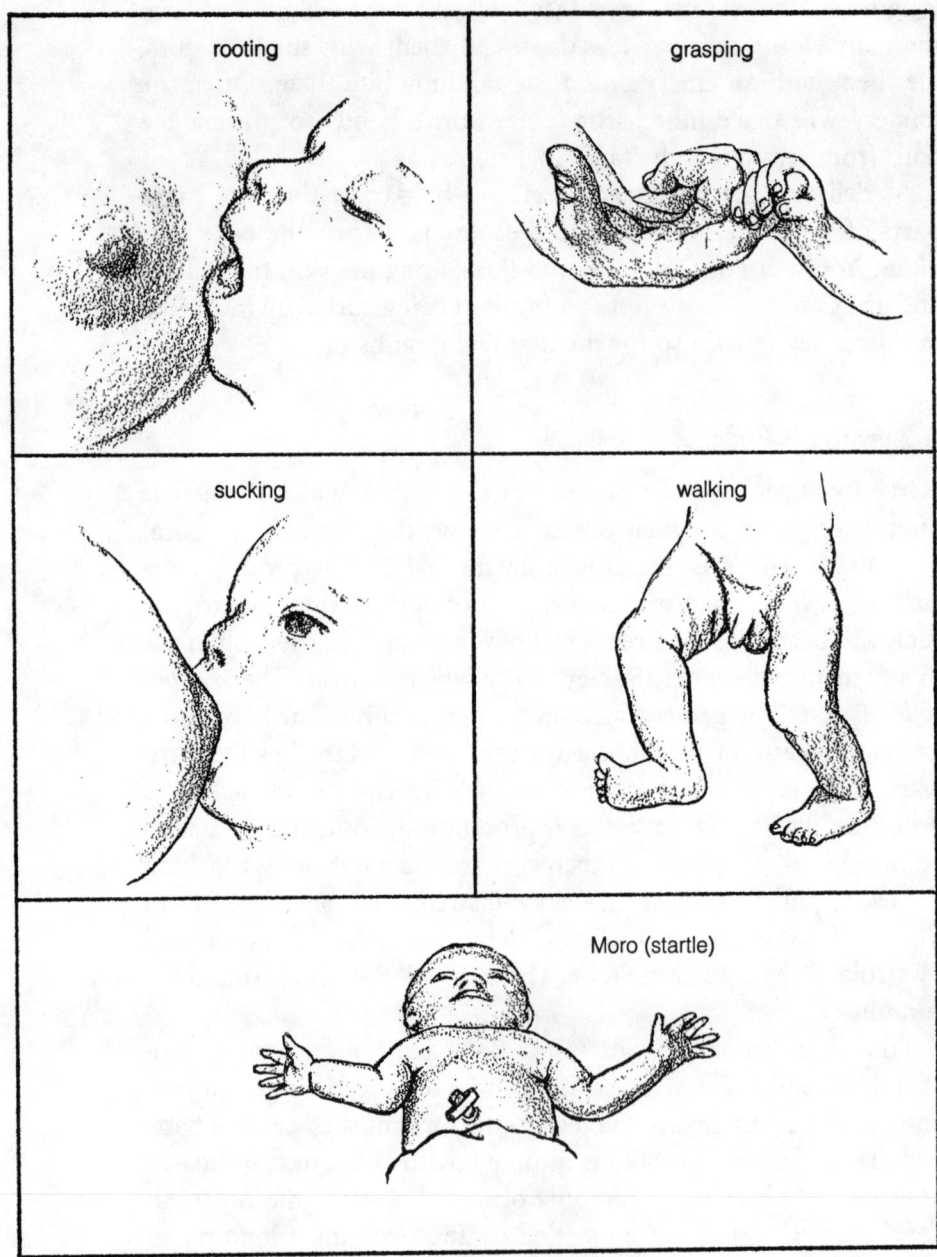

rooting

grasping

sucking

walking

Moro (startle)

Fig. 52. The reflexes of a newborn.

Circumcision

Circumcision is the surgical removal of the foreskin covering the penis of male babies. It has been a widespread practice in the United States for the last 40 years. The American Academy of Pediatrics recently stated that they consider it a nonessential surgical procedure, because it offers no health benefits that can't be obtained by good personal hygiene. If your baby is a boy, you will be asked to decide whether or not you want him circumcised.

Some facts you might want to know about circumcision are as follows:

- Circumcision does not prevent cancer of the penis.
- Circumcision will not prevent cervical cancer in future sexual partners.
- There is no relationship between circumcision and sexual pleasure.
- Circumcision will not prevent masturbation.

Most physicians give the following three reasons for circumcision: (1) A circumcised penis may be easier to keep clean. (2) In certain religious groups, including Jews and Moslems, circumcision is a required ritual. (3) If other men in the family are circumcised, the boy will look more like them.

Reasons against circumcision are as follows: (1) It is unnecessary surgery, with risks of bleeding and infection. (2) Proper hygiene can prevent infection in later life, just as circumcision does. (3) The baby feels pain, although we do not know how much.

If your baby is circumcised, the area will need to be kept clean in the few days it takes to heal. After circumcision, a piece of gauze dipped in petroleum jelly will be placed loosely around the tip of the penis. Changing the gauze with each diaper change will prevent infection. If you notice the penis becoming swollen, or if it bleeds, contact the baby's health-care provider.

Problems of Newborns

Most newborns are born without complications and go home with mother at her discharge from the hospital, but some encounter problems and need to stay in the hospital for observation or treatment. Below are some of the conditions that might keep your child in the hospital.

Jaundice. Jaundice is a yellowish discoloration of the skin caused by bilirubin, a product of the breakdown of red blood cells. All newborns make bilirubin, though some make more than others, and all newborns have difficulty removing bilirubin from the blood stream during the first few days. A number of healthy babies will become jaundiced around the second or third day of life. The jaundice is entirely harmless and fades in the first week of life.

Jaundice can have many other causes, however, such as lack of certain enzymes, prematurity, infection, and dehydration. Jaundice can also be a sign that there is a difference between the blood types of mother and baby, called ABO incompatibility or Rh incompatibility. ABO incompatibility is less serious than Rh disease and more common; both can cause jaundice because antibodies made by the mother destroy red blood cells in the baby. Other rare causes include a congenital obstruction of the flow of bile through the liver or gall bladder and viruses that result in certain types of hepatitis.

Severe jaundice can cause brain damage, so physicians will treat the condition if it worsens. The most common treatment is placing the baby under ultraviolet light, which breaks down bilirubin in the baby's skin. Babies under ultraviolet light need extra fluid and sometimes are irritable, but this therapy is quite effective and safe. If ultraviolet treatment is not successful, then an exchange transfusion, which removes a small amount of the baby's blood and bilirubin, and replaces it with fresh blood, will bring the bilirubin down to a safe level.

Prematurity. Babies born before 37 weeks experience a number of problems directly related to their age at birth. They are smaller, skinnier, and have less body than full-term infants. Many premature babies have trouble breathing regularly or efficiently and require oxygen or a machine to help them breathe until they become strong enough to do so effectively on their own. They are also less able to maintain their body temperature and require constant warming in an isolette, or incubator. Babies born before 35 weeks of age often have trouble sucking and have to be fed through small feeding tubes placed from the mouth or nose into the stomach. Premature infants may also suffer from jaundice and hypoglycemia (low blood sugar). Infants less than 34 weeks may develop respiratory distress syndrome, a condition where the lungs cannot fully expand with oxygen.

Babies weighing less than four-and-a-half pounds or arriving before 36 weeks are usually placed in an intensive care nursery for observation and to be given the extra attention and care they require. Most intensive care nurseries have 24-hour visiting for parents, and many mothers of premature babies breastfeed babies with the encouragement of the nursery staff. If your premature baby cannot be breastfed, you can pump your breast milk, which will be fed to your baby by tube. Most hospitals will discharge healthy premature infants when they reach four-and-a-half or five pounds.

Postmature Babies. Occasionally a pregnancy continues past 42 weeks. By the time of delivery, the baby has long fingernails and very creased skin, which is thick and may have already begun to peel. A postmature infant may have also already passed meconium into the amniotic fluid while still in the uterus, which can cause problems with breathing after delivery and may stain the skin and umbilical cord yellow. Often, postmature infants have trouble feeding and appear restless and unusually hungry.

Twins. About one birth in 100 is twin delivery. Triplets occur once in every 8,000 births, and quadruplets only once in every 700,000 births. With the increased use of fertility drugs, multiple births have become more common. Today, health-care providers identify twins before delivery. There remain special risks that may accompany multiple births, such as premature labor, breech presentation, and unequal nutrition of the babies. Often, twin infants are smaller and suffer from the same problems as premature infants.

Feeding Your Baby

Breast or bottle? Which is best? There are advantages and disadvantages to each. How you decide to feed your baby will depend on many factors including how you were fed as a baby, how your friends feed their babies, what your work schedule and time constraints are, whether the baby will be in daycare or not, and the advice you receive from your midwife or physician. The American Academy of Pediatrics, as well as almost all international associations concerned with children's health, recommends breastfeeding as the preferred way to feed an infant. The box on the next page lists some pros and cons for both methods.

Many parents combine breast- and bottle-feeding with excellent results. This is often the method of choice for working mothers, who cannot be available 24 hours a day to feed their babies. Working mothers will often breastfeed two or three times a day and give

Breastfeeding/Bottle-feeding

Advantages of Breastfeeding

Human milk is the perfect food for the newborn, containing the right nutrients in the right proportions.

Colostrum, the watery fluid in the breast during the first few days after delivery, contains antibodies and proteins that protect babies from a wide variety of diseases and helps clear meconium from the infant's intestinal tract.

Breast milk is easier for the newborn to digest than cow's milk.

There are no known allergies to breast milk.

Breast milk is cheaper than formula. It requires no storage, cannot spoil, and is always ready for baby.

You can freeze breast milk and defrost it as you need it for bottle-feeds.

There is less chance of overfeeding with breastfeeding.

Breastfed babies tend to have less diarrhea, or vomiting, and tend to swallow less air than bottle-fed babies.

Advantages of Bottle-feeding

Mother does not have to be present to feed the baby. Father can be equally involved with the feeding of the infant.

As it is more difficult for a baby to digest cow's milk, a bottle-fed baby may sleep longer than a breastfed baby.

Parents can be assured of how much their baby is eating.

Commercial formulas may be more expensive but are convenient, available, easy to prepare, and easily transportable.

Parents may feel more comfortable feeding their babies in public.

Bottle-feeding requires less of a time commitment from the mother, allowing her more freedom with her schedule; the father or other family members can become involved more easily in the child's care.

Bottle-feeding is easier in the beginning with the first child, requiring less instruction and support from health-care providers or family.

the baby pumped breast milk or formula for the other feeds. Many parents work out a system that suits the individual situation.

In deciding how to feed your child, do what is best for you. Remember, however, that breastfeeding for even a short while gives your baby important protection against certain infections, and can be a very emotionally gratifying experience.

RECOMMENDED RESOURCES

Behrman, Richard E., and Victor C. Vaughn. *Nelson Textbook of Pediatrics*. Philadelphia: W. B. Saunders Company, 1983. The definitive pediatric textbook, used as a resource by most pediatric health-care providers.

Chess, Stella, Thomas Alexander, and Herbert Birch. *Your Child Is a Person*. New York: Viking Press, 1965. The first book that explained differences in children's temperament from birth on. An important work on child development and behavior.

Queenan, John, ed. *A New Life: Pregnancy, Birth, and Your Child's First Year*. New York: Van Nostrand Reinhold Company, 1979. A comprehensive book about the entire experience of pregnancy, delivery, and the first year of life. A good reference book for both health-care providers and mothers.

25 Basic Training for New Parents

After surviving labor and delivery, the next test of parenthood is learning how to take care of a new baby. If you have not been a parent of an infant or had experience taking care of a newborn, being responsible for the well-being of a tiny baby can seem overwhelming. Many new parents get home and suddenly realize that in spite of all of the books they have read, movies they have watched, and classes they have attended, they do not know how to take care of, hold, diaper, or feed their new baby.

In those first few days at home, your baby will be your teacher, telling you with its cry when it is hungry, wet, or frustrated. The cry is a signal that the baby needs something, be it comfort, food, or attention. You will learn quickly what to do. After you have satisfied its physical needs, hold and rock your baby. The physical closeness may be just what the newborn needs to calm down and prepare for sleep.

There is no right way to diaper, nurse, burp, dress, or wrap a baby. Find the methods that work for you. Here are a few handy self-preservation tricks: quiet an infant by placing your little finger in its mouth to let it suck, pat a baby's back if a burp is long in coming, and rub the newborn's back when it is fussy, and hold an infant by supporting its head (see fig. 53). When changing a diaper, have a clean one handy so something absorbent can be placed quickly over the baby's bare bottom. Each time you figure out what your baby needs and satisfy that need, you will have another bit of information about your baby. The next time you get that same signal, you will know what it means.

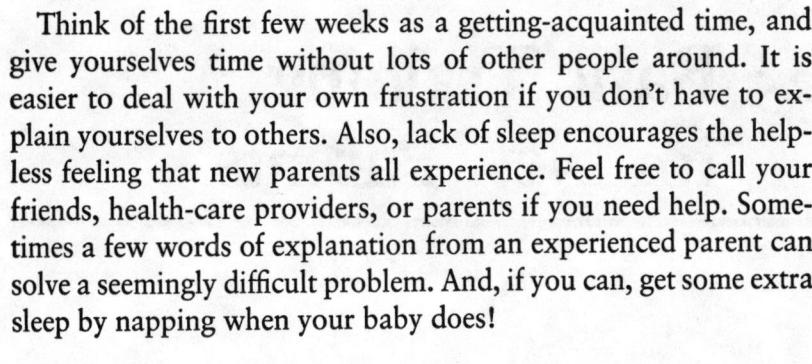

Think of the first few weeks as a getting-acquainted time, and give yourselves time without lots of other people around. It is easier to deal with your own frustration if you don't have to explain yourselves to others. Also, lack of sleep encourages the helpless feeling that new parents all experience. Feel free to call your friends, health-care providers, or parents if you need help. Sometimes a few words of explanation from an experienced parent can solve a seemingly difficult problem. And, if you can, get some extra sleep by napping when your baby does!

Fig. 53. A safe, comfortable way to hold a baby.

Nursing: How to Do It

Your baby is born with many instinctive reflexes, the ability to suck being the most important one for survival. A lot of mothers assume that their babies will begin to suck when first given the breast; however, many babies are too tired to nurse after delivery. It doesn't hurt to put your newborn to the breast anyway. He or she may suck for a few seconds and become more alert, or continue to be drowsy. Some infants have less developed sucking reflexes, which makes it difficult for both mother and baby. Even a hungry baby can have difficulty finding the breast. Don't be discouraged if your infant is a slow starter. He or she won't be for long! Successful breastfeeding is a learned skill for both mother and baby.

The first thing to do is get in a comfortable position. You can nurse sitting up or lying down (fig. 54), or in whatever position you find best for you. Many new mothers find sitting to be the most comfortable position during the first few days of breastfeeding. If you are sitting, support a straight back with a few pillows, and place the baby on a pillow on your lap. You can then position your knees to bring the baby closer to your breast and move him or her in a way that brings the nipple into contact with the baby's mouth. Some mothers find that using a pillow to support the arm in which the baby lies will keep the arm from aching. If your baby's cheek is against your breast and its legs are underneath your opposite arm, you are in a position for nursing.

If you are lying down, try lying on your side with a few pillows behind your back and one underneath your head. Support the infant's head with a folded diaper as he or she lies close to you; this

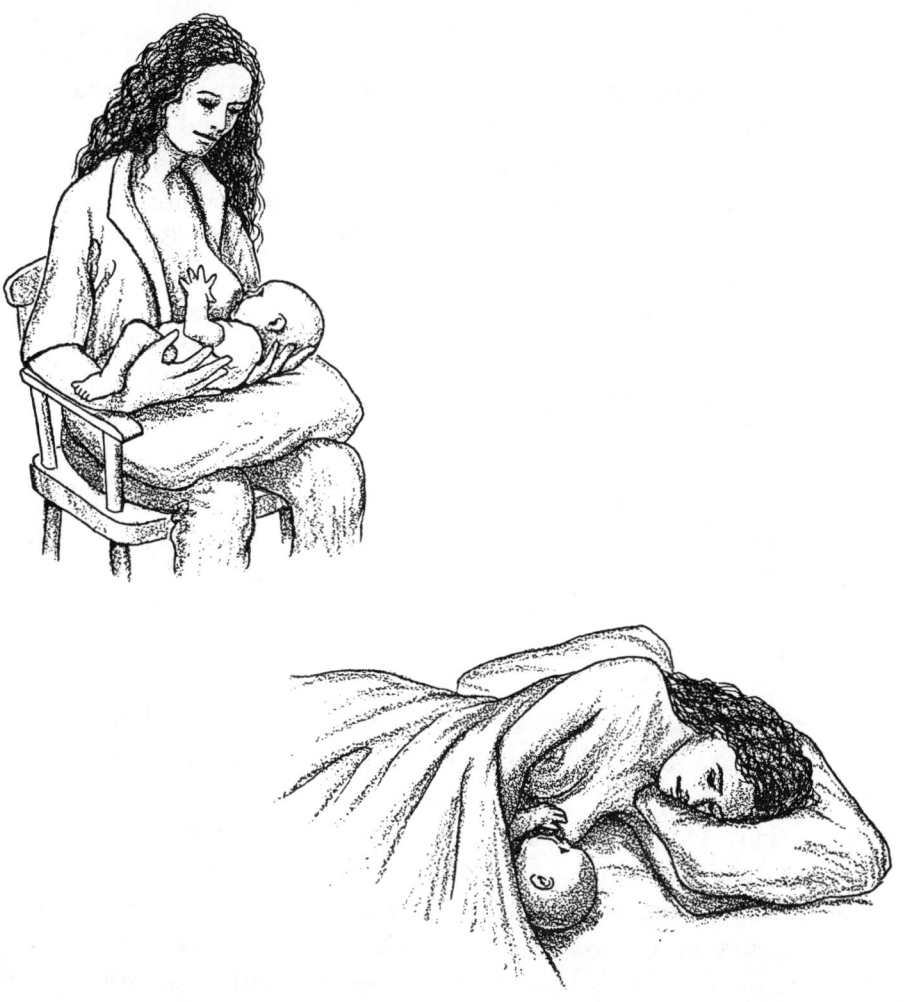

Fig. 54. Two comfortable positions for breastfeeding.

will position its head near the nipple. The familiar rocking chair provides a rhythm that seems just right for breastfeeding a hungry baby.

The next task is getting your baby on the breast. It's of the utmost importance that your baby take the entire areola (pigmented part) of the nipple into its mouth: getting the baby on your nipple properly can prevent sore nipples and can make the milk flow well. Your baby is born with a rooting reflex that turns his or her head toward anything that remotely resembles a nipple. Try stroking the baby's cheek or nuzzling his or her face in your breast until he or she turns toward the nipple. Then, help your baby grab onto your nipple and areola by holding your breast between your thumb and forefinger. If the baby grabs onto the nipple only, take him or her off the breast and begin again. You can lightly touch the nipple against the baby's lips to open its mouth wide enough to take in the entire nipple and areola. It is the up-and-down motion of the infant's mouth that compresses the areola and begins the release of milk. The placement of the baby's tongue underneath the nipple also helps push the milk out. The nipple needs to be drawn back into the baby's mouth for this to happen. Mothers with especially large or engorged breasts may need to place a finger between the base of the nipple and the baby's mouth to allow the baby to get air through his or her nose. This is important to remember since a newborn does not know how to breathe through its mouth. When it is time to take the baby off the breast, gently break the suction by sliding a finger inside its mouth. If you try to pull your baby off your nipple, he or she will immediately clamp down and tighten the grip on your nipple, leaving you sore and in pain.

Most mothers offer each breast at each feeding. The first breast offered usually empties more, so you may want to alternate breasts at each new feeding, beginning with the last breast offered at the previous feed. You can keep track of which breast was last given by pinning a safety pin to the nursing bra on the side last given, moving the safety pin after each feeding.

How long should you nurse on each side? This depends on you and the condition of your nipples. In the first few days of breast-feeding, some women get very sore nipples from even short periods of nursing. The average time that seems to work for most women on the first day is about five minutes on each breast, with a good burp in between. Increase to seven to ten minutes the next day, and finally to fifteen minutes, or whatever time your baby needs to feed after that. Nursing for less then three minutes on a side, especially in the beginning, prevents the let-down reflex (emptying of the breast) from developing appropriately; long periods of nursing leave the mother with very sore nipples. Once you have been nursing for a while and your let-down reflex is well established, your baby should get most of the milk it needs in the first five minutes of nursing.

Breastfed babies swallow less air than bottle-fed babies, but they still need to be burped to release the air swallowed during a feed. Some babies hardly burp, while others let out a hearty noise with each burp. Both are normal. The best time to burp is after you have given one breast. The three most common positions for burping are placing the baby over your shoulder, sitting the baby up in your lap while supporting its head, or laying the baby over your knees. Patting the baby's back lightly, or rubbing its back, usually results in a good burp. If no burp occurs after a few minutes, give your baby the other breast and then try burping again after you have finished feeding.

Most mothers need three or four nursing bras. To absorb the leaking milk, you can buy disposable nursing pads or insert pieces of soft cotton to protect your nipples from getting sore. Old handkerchiefs or pieces of T-shirts or sweatshirt material make great nursing pads and can be cut to size and washed regularly. Leaking is common in the first few weeks as the let-down reflex is established but disappears in the first few months. If it continues to be a problem, you can wear a tighter bra or compress your breast with your arm when you feel the tingling of the let-down reflex begin.

Many mothers prefer to wear button-front blouses or dresses, or knit pullovers, which allow you to nurse without exposing your breast. Scarves or shawls draped across your breasts provide ways to breastfeed in public places without showing a bare midriff. Some mothers create ingenious garments with hidden zippers, pockets across the breasts that lift up, or large collars that can be removed to make breastfeeding more convenient.

Bottle-feeding: How to Do It

For those who decide to bottle-feed, three questions often come up: Which formula do I give my baby? Do I have to sterilize the bottles? And, how much do I feed my baby? Your health-care provider will suggest which formula to use. Often, the hospital will give you a free starter kit of the formula the baby was fed in the hospital, and if this formula agrees with your newborn, stick with it. There are three or four major brands of cow's-milk-based formula in the United States today, and all are available in supermarkets and pharmacies. If you think your child is having problems with the formula, consult your pediatrician or family physician before changing brands. Many prepared formulas come packaged in pre-filled bottles, or eight-ounce ready-to-serve cans. However, they are less expensive if purchased in large quart cans, which come both as ready-to-serve or as concentrate, to which you just add water.

You will need about eight to twelve bottles in all, either glass or plastic, each of which holds a minimum of four ounces of milk. It is important to buy the nipples, caps, and collars that specifically fit your bottles. If you buy the bottles with disposable plastic liners, buy enough liners for eight feeds a day. Most nipples have up and down sides, and are shaped to fit into the baby's mouth a certain way.

Although bottles do not necessarily need to be sterilized, they should be kept very clean. Even if you have a dishwasher, a good bottle brush is handy for removing dried bits of milk from hard-to-reach places.

Start with a clean bottle, nipple, collar, and cap. Use a clean can opener to open the formula can, and carefully measure out concentrated formula with the proper measuring cups. Put the appropriate amount of formula into each bottle; if a concentrate is used, dilute with boiled water. Put the nipples, collars, and caps on each bottle and store them in the refrigerator to be used within 24 hours. Some parents close the tops loosely, put the bottles into a sterilizer or large pot, boil them for 20 minutes, cool them for two hours, and then place them in a refrigerator with tightened caps. The boiling allows the milk to be used for a 48-hour period. Label the bottles with the time and dates so you know when they need to be thrown out. If you have any doubts about the freshness of the formula, toss it out. If your baby does not finish a bottle within two hours, throw it out; refrigerating it again will not prevent contamination by bacteria.

A new baby will drink between two and five ounces per feed during the first few weeks. Before long, you will recognize a regular daily feeding pattern, with the amount differing depending on the time of day and the baby's growth spurts. A feed can take up to 20 minutes. If it takes longer, check to see whether the nipple's hole is too small, or whether there are lots of air bubbles in the bottle.

While giving the bottle, hold your baby in the crook of your elbow, supporting its head and neck (see fig. 55). Make eye contact, and keep the baby's head higher than its stomach. Never prop up the bottle and leave the baby, who might gag or choke. If the milk is coming out too fast or too slowly, adjust the collar around the nipple and check the hole size. If you can't adjust the flow, new nipples may be needed. Burp the baby once every two ounces unless you find that burping that often is not needed. Some mothers heat formula, but it is not necessary to do so. Room temperature is fine. Remember that giving a bottle to your baby is providing it with love as well as food, and that feeding times are special times for parents as well as babies.

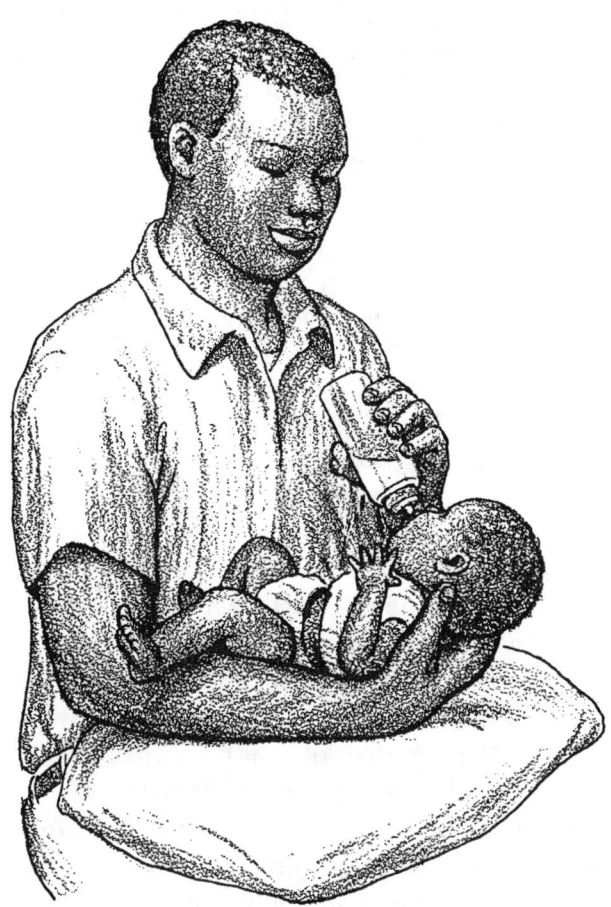

Fig. 55. A comfortable way to bottle-feed.

How Often Should You Feed Your Infant?

How often you feed your infant depends on you and your infant. Many mothers feed on demand for the first few weeks until the baby establishes a regular feeding schedule. Demand feeding is the easiest way to assure yourself that your baby is getting enough food. For the breastfeeding mother, however, demand feeding can be uncomfortable if the baby feeds continually. Both bottle-feeding and breastfeeding mothers find that feeding every two to three hours for the first weeks helps to establish a feeding schedule they can live with.

By the time your baby is six weeks old, you will have a good idea what the cry of hunger sounds like. Most likely your infant will have established a feeding schedule. Feeding every two or every four hours may be normal for your baby. If you are worried that your baby is not getting enough food, or getting too much food, you can buy a kitchen scale (up to 25 lbs.) and weigh your baby daily. Steady weight gain is a good sign, but contact your health-care provider if your infant loses weight.

Bathing Your Baby

Bathing a newborn is not necessary every day. Usually, a couple of baths a week are enough. Wiping the baby's skin with a soft cotton towel dampened with warm water, and then drying with a dry towel, is all your little one needs during the first days.

Within a few days, you can proceed to a formal sponge bath. A sponge bath can be used anytime you don't wish to bother with a tub bath. Some physicians recommend these sponge or towel baths until the umbilical cord stump falls off. To give a sponge bath, use warm water and a very mild soap (Dove is the mildest on the market), with a soft washcloth or a small bath sponge. Sponge off, soap, and then rinse one part of your baby's body at a time; if the room is cool, you may want to dry the clean part off right away. Be sure to wipe all the creases and folds of your baby's skin. Don't use soap on the face. Instead, use warm water, wiping the eyes from the center outwards with a clean washcloth or damp cotton balls to prevent infection. Avoid using cotton applicators in the nostrils or ears, but use them to clean around the umbilical stump daily.

Once the cord is off and the stump has healed, your baby will be ready for a tub bath (fig. 56). Choose a container that suits your needs. A plastic dishpan is cheap and safe, stores easily, and can be run through the dishwasher when dirty. Fill the tub with a small amount of warm water. Arrange the bath paraphernalia so you do not have to let go of the baby during the bath. Hold the baby in a comfortable way that allows you to have a secure grip. Wash and rinse each part as you do when giving a sponge bath. Afterwards, place the baby in a soft warm towel and dry carefully the creases and folds of skin to prevent irritation. As your baby gets older, he or she can bathe with you in the tub; it's a lot of fun. Most little ones begin to splash and kick and find bath time a treat. Many working fathers find that bath time is a good way for them to relax with their babies after a long workday.

Like bathing, shampooing is not required for a baby. To shampoo your baby's head, use a bit of soap or baby shampoo, or just

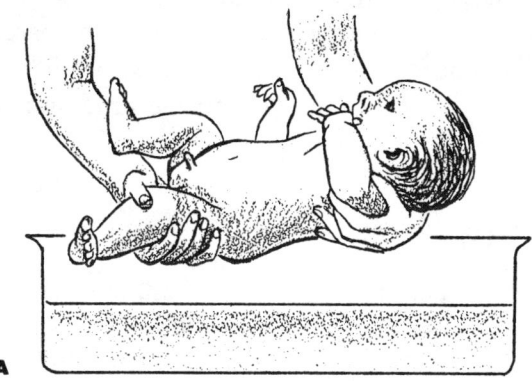

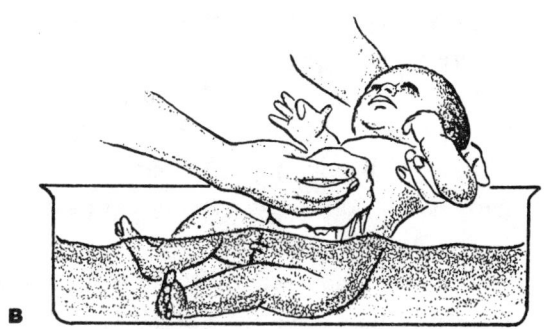

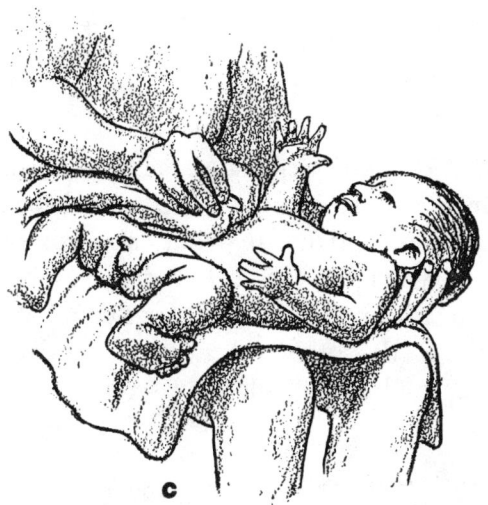

Fig. 56. Bathing and drying off your baby. (A) Support the head and hips before placing baby in water. (B) Do not submerge baby; support the head while sponging each body part individually. (C) Be sure to dry off each crease well with a soft towel to prevent skin irritation.

use clear water. Rinse the head carefully, pouring water toward the baby's back to prevent getting shampoo in the eyes. Many parents use a cup to rinse off the head. This allows you to use one hand to support the baby's head while rinsing. Dry off the head and ears carefully.

Care of the Umbilical Cord Stump

The stump of the umbilical cord will dry up and fall off within the first two weeks. Until it does, clean it with a cotton swab dipped in alcohol. When the stump comes off, a small raw area will be left exposed where the cord attached to the skin. This spot usually heals very quickly. Fold the diaper down to keep the area uncovered and to promote healing.

There may be a slight discharge from the healing umbilical cord. Clean it off with alcohol. If a discharge persists for more than a few days, ask your pediatrician or family physician to see your baby. Occasionally, a baby develops an infection that needs to be treated with antibiotics.

The umbilicus usually retracts after the cord remnant falls off, creating a navel that goes inwards. A few remain outward, but neither type causes problems. There is not much parents can do to influence whether the navel heals in or out.

Changing Your Baby

With the advent of disposable diapers, changing the baby has become a skill that takes little time to learn. Most parents become experts while still at the hospital, and you and your baby will soon find a system that works for you both. Using cloth diapers takes a little more skill but can also be learned quickly. Change your baby's diaper as often as he or she needs it; this will prevent most diaper rashes. Remember to clean and dry off the baby's bottom well. Here are a few hints:

- Have everything in reach before you begin the diaper change (fig. 57), including cotton or diaper wipes to clean off the baby's bottom. Don't leave your baby unattended on the changing table.
- Many babies, especially boy babies, pee in the middle of a diaper change. Have a clean diaper or towel in hand to prevent a spray or puddle.
- If you are using cloth diapers, use a bar of soap or a sponge to stick the pins into while changing the diaper.

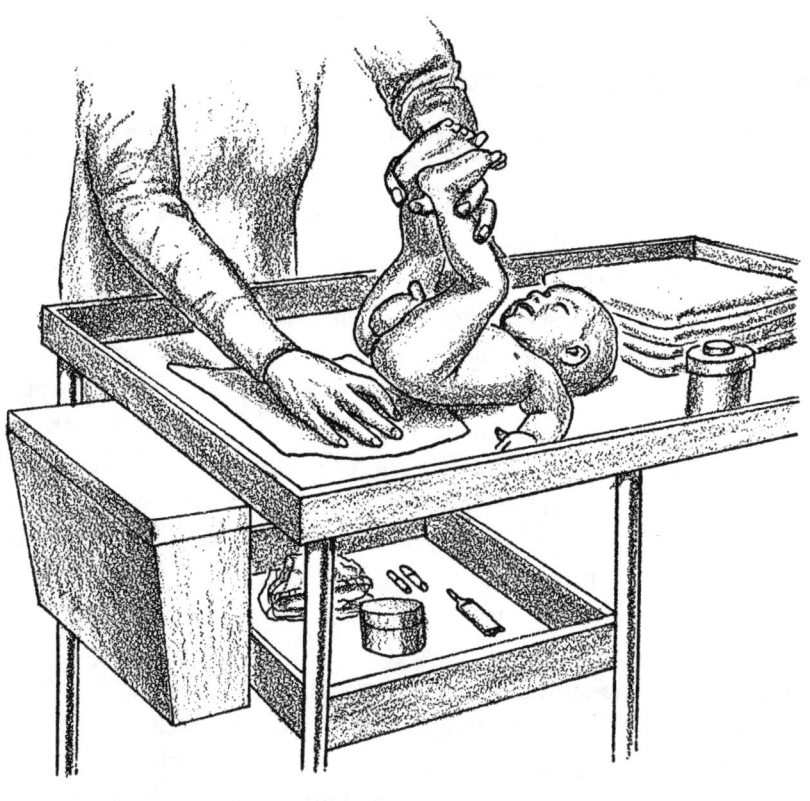

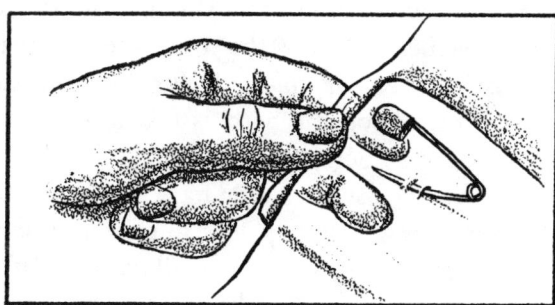

Fig. 57. Changing your baby. When pinning a diaper, place your hand between the baby's skin and the diaper.

• If you are pinning a diaper, protect your baby from puncture by placing your hand in between the baby's skin and the diaper. You can use plastic diaper pins or diaper clips as a safeguard.

• The diaper, either cloth or paper, should fit snugly around the baby's legs to prevent leakage, but not tightly enough to leave marks on the baby's legs or to cause irritation.

• If you use disposable diapers, buy the ones with reusable tapes. If the tape loses its stick, you can still use the diaper by using extra adhesive tape to close the diaper.

Bowel Movements and Urination

While still in the uterus, your baby passed urine into the amniotic fluid, beginning very early in the pregnancy. Shortly after birth, most babies urinate. Thereafter, the amount of urination depends on how much fluid the baby drinks. For the first few days, babies may only pee three or four times a day, increasing to up to ten times a day by the first week of life. Urination usually accompanies a bowel movement. The color of the urine depends on the amount of water in it and how much a baby has been drinking. If your baby's urine is quite dark, he or she may need to drink more often.

Stools vary in color and consistency depending on whether your baby is breast- or bottle-fed. In the first 24 hours after delivery, the baby will pass a sticky, dark-green meconium stool. During the first few days at home, the stools will change in color and consistency. Breastfed babies pass yellow stools, often like cottage cheese in consistency and slightly sweet smelling, between three and six times a day. The stools of bottle-fed babies are paler and have a stronger odor. The consistency is usually harder and grittier, more like clay. Bottle-fed babies have less frequent bowel movements, one to three a day on average. Some babies will have bowel movements after every feed, while others will skip a day and then have two consecutive movements. Unless the stools are very watery, or very hard, there is no need for alarm. Color and consistency of stools will vary with the food the baby is fed. If you have questions, contact your baby's doctor for help.

If you notice that your baby is passing hard stools, whether you are bottle- or breastfeeding, you may need to give your baby more water. Hard stools occasionally cause a small amount of bleeding from the rectum. If this occurs, talk the situation over with your pediatrician or family physician.

Sleep and the Lack of It

Most parents are exhausted by the time the mother and child come home from the hospital. The labor and delivery, the excitement of the new baby, and unfamiliar hospital routines prevent mothers from getting enough sleep. Fathers get little rest after the delivery, calling friends and relatives, taking care of other children, or staying at the hospital. The new arrival then comes home, and mother and father get even more tired meeting the needs of the new infant. When mother is overtired, she eats less and drinks less, which can slow healing and decrease breast-milk production. Lack of sleep also intensifies emotional fluctuations of the first days of the post-partum period, and can lead to depression.

After the intense experience of a delivery, some parents feel let down. Because of changes in hormone levels, many mothers experience mood swings. What does this all add up to? Irritability, fatigue, and depression? Not necessarily. New parents can combat this exhaustion by limiting visitors and extra activities in the first few weeks after delivery. Sleep is a much-needed medicine for both parents and baby. It replenishes both physically and emotionally and allows the new family some time alone.

Your Other Children

When baby makes four, five, or six in a family, parents are faced with new challenges. Most children look forward to the birth of a new sibling, with the older children making the adjustment to a new family member more easily than toddlers. A six-year-old can clearly see how he or she can be mother's helper where a toddler is not able to take on the role of the older sibling with as much understanding. Most of the negative behavior an older child exhibits will be directed at mother.

Parents may feel anxious or guilty about having to divide their attention between the older child and the infant, but they are likely to feel guiltier when their older child shows resentment toward the new baby. These guilt feelings are natural and are experienced by all parents in varying degrees.

Most experts agree that older children will adjust more easily if they are involved in preparations for the baby, and if ways are found for them to help out once the baby arrives. Take them with you to your prenatal visits and let them hear the fetal heartbeat. If they can be present when the baby is born, the experience will help them bond with their new sibling. If they cannot be there, explain to your children what will happen when you go to the hospital, and tell them ahead of time who will be taking care of them in your absence. It helps to have a present for your older children from the new baby on your return from the hospital; this makes them feel that the baby wants to be loved by them. If you have a toddler, give him or her a new doll to play "baby" with. Your child can then act out some hostility on the doll, not the new infant. If possible, let the older children help care for the new baby, pointing out how grown up they are by letting them select the clothing or the diaper that the new baby will wear. Finally, let your children know that they are loved by setting aside time to spend exclusively with them.

Some parents feel that it takes longer for them to bond with their second or third child. Often the intensity of the emotional experience of birth is greatest with the first delivery, and is lessened subsequently. In addition, having another child who needs attention and love makes the parents unable to devote their attention and feelings exclusively to the new baby. If you find it taking longer than you expect to feel close to your second child, don't feel guilty; it is normal. Try to be relaxed, and allow time for the new arrival to become part of the family.

Visitors

For new parents who are physically tired from labor and delivery, or from adjusting to the birth of a new baby, constant visitors can be a major source of stress and conflict. In the hospital, visiting hours are restricted and in most rooming-in situations, only fathers, grandparents, and siblings are allowed to visit. Some health-care providers send their patients home with a family prescription limiting visitors and family to a 15-minute visit around 5:00 P.M. This prescription then permits the family to limit or extend the visit as they choose, using the health-care provider's prescription as a reason to cut short a visit if desired. Some friends will come for a short visit, bring dinner for the new family, and leave before their welcome is spent. However, you may need to ask others to leave so you can get the sleep and time alone you need. Sleep when your baby is sleeping, so you can be fresh and ready for the next feeding.

One kind of visitor can be a tremendous help and, if available, should be welcomed: a close relative (usually a grandmother of the new baby) who comes for a few days or weeks to help out.

Getting on a Schedule

Though it may seem at first that there isn't a pattern or routine that fits your baby's sleep and wake time, within the first few weeks most parents and babies settle down to a routine that revolves around feeding times. Many parents find that their babies wake around a certain time and require food or comfort at the same times each day. Learning the difference between cries for comfort, food, or attention will help you settle into a routine at home. If the baby is bottle-fed, father or older siblings can often help out mother with the feeds, freeing up some time for her. Mother naturally has to handle breastfeeding, but dad can then take over nonfeeding activities, such as bathing, diapering, or soothing a fussy little one. Often, newborns are consoled just by being bundled up and placed against a parent's chest or abdomen.

Parents should try to modify their household chores for the first weeks until a routine of sleeping and waking is established. (A baby carrier comes in handy and allows you to have both hands free.) Some creative parents use paper plates and eat frozen dinners until things are more in control. Instead of cooking and cleaning up, they sleep. Accept offers of help from friends and relatives: a good friend will realize that doing your laundry is of more value than taking you out to lunch.

RECOMMENDED RESOURCES

Eiger, Marvin, and Sally Wendkos Olds. *The Complete Book of Breastfeeding.* New York: Workman Publishing Company, 1972. A how-to book that answers all your questions about breastfeeding.

Kitzinger, Sheila. *The Experience of Breastfeeding.* Harmondsworth, England, and New York: Penguin Books, 1979. In this companion to her book *The Experience of Childbirth*, Sheila Kitzinger tells in poetic prose what breastfeeding is all about.

La Leche League International. *The Womanly Art of Breastfeeding.* New York: New American Library, 1981. The La Leche Bible—this book tells you what to do and why. Some women find this book a little preachy, but it's full of good information and support for breastfeeders.

Mueser, Anne Marie, and George Verrilli. *Welcome Baby: A Guide to the First Six Weeks.* New York: St. Martin's Press, 1982. An easy-to-read glossary on everything you want to know about a new baby.

26 Problems with Your Baby

It is normal for parents, especially new parents, to get anxious when their infant is sick. Babies are helpless and unable to tell their parents what is wrong with them. They send signals that often are confusing to the most experienced pediatrician. However, there are some problems you should be able to recognize and know whether they warrant immediate attention.

Five problems you should particularly worry about in your newborn are dehydration, diarrhea, fever, lethargy or inability to arouse your baby, and vomiting. Any of these problems may indicate that your infant is ill and may need to see a doctor. Often a change in behavior will be your baby's signal that he or she is sick. The baby's routine will change, and you may notice more fussiness, less interest in eating, or some other change in activity.

If you think your baby is sick, seek professional advice. Often you can get reassurance from your doctor as he or she answers your questions about your baby's behavior or symptoms. Doctors understand that parents may have lots of questions about their baby's health in the first few months. If an infant is ill, they expect to be awakened at night. It is better to call when you are worried at night than to wait eight hours and bring a very sick baby to the doctor in the morning.

A Glossary of Concerns

Choking. Sometimes while feeding, your baby will start to choke. If this happens, hold the baby face down, head lower than the body, and pat the baby's back gently. Usually, the baby will then regurgitate some of the milk, cough a few times, and resume breathing without difficulty.

Colic. Colic is a term used to describe attacks of fussiness, crying, and abdominal pain, supposedly of intestinal origin. It affects many infants under three months of age. An attack usually begins with loud and continuous crying. The baby's stomach may distend and he or she may grimace and pull the legs up. The crying attack can last for hours, sometimes ending when the baby passes stool or falls asleep.

Parents of "colicky" infants must use extra effort to calm their infants. Some successful techniques include swaddling your infant, placing the infant in a swing (with the rocking motion continued until the baby quiets), walking the baby around, going for a car ride, and placing the baby in its car seat on top of a dryer filled with towels which cause the dryer to vibrate, thus soothing the infant. Overfeeding, or feeding too frequently, may worsen the crying attacks. The attacks almost always begin to lessen by three months of age (just when parents have reached the end of their rope!).

Constipation. Practically unknown in breastfed babies, and rare in bottle-fed babies, constipation in an infant is the passage of hard-formed stools. Some babies on formulas with iron supplementation have harder stools. In warm weather, constipation can indicate the need for additional fluid; try giving the infant more water. If the condition persists, consult your physician before changing the baby's diet.

Cradle-Cap. This is a flaky or crusty formation on the top of an infant's head. It develops from dried oil and dead skin, which build up to form a crust. Parents can get rid of cradle-cap by gently washing the baby's head with baby shampoo, loosening the crust, and then combing it out of the hair. Applying baby oil to the scalp a day before shampooing helps dissolve the oils in cradle-cap by moisturizing the skin. If the baby's scalp appears red or begins to ooze a clear fluid, contact the baby's doctor for advice.

Crying. Crying is the way your new infant tells you that it needs something. It is then up to you to figure out what the baby needs and how to satisfy it. After a few days with their newborn, many parents can distinguish a cry of hunger from a cry for comfort.

However, even experienced parents often go through trial and error before they figure out what a baby wants. Consider all of the reasons that may cause your infant to cry—including hunger, thirst, need for diaper change, need to suck, uncomfortable positioning, desire to be touched, need to be comforted, need for sleep, need for burping, excessive warmth, not enough warmth, and others. Most of the time you can provide your child with the comfort it needs.

Dehydration. Dehydration, or excessive loss of body water, is usually caused by severe diarrhea or vomiting or by not drinking enough fluids. Children and adults can lose quite a lot of water before becoming dehydrated; but because infants have so little extra body fluid, they can become dehydrated quickly. Thus a newborn can become dehydrated within 12 hours if he or she is not able to drink fluids or is losing a lot of fluid in diarrheal stools. Signs of dehydration in an infant are weight loss, decreased urination, doughy skin, sunken eyes or a sunken anterior fontanelle, decreased tears, and a dry mouth. Infants who are dehydrated are often restless, irritable, or drowsy. If you think your baby has any of these signs or symptoms, call your doctor immediately.

Diaper Rash. Three kinds of diaper rash plague infants: (1) The ammonical rash, usually from the ammonia in the urine. This can be cleared up by keeping baby's bottom dry, sometimes letting it air-dry without a diaper for periods of time. (2) A monilial diaper rash, caused by the fungus *Candida*. It looks red and irritated, and may require a medicated cream to clear up. (3) Seborrheic diaper rash, which is dry and crusted, often oozing clear fluid. It may also require medicated creams to clear up.

Help prevent diaper rash by cleaning the area well at diaper changes, changing the diaper more often, and not using rubber pants with cloth diapers. A&D ointment, Desitin, or Diaperene cream may help protect your baby's bottom and can treat mild rashes. Corn starch is an excellent powder to use with each diaper change; it absorbs moisture and helps prevent rashes.

Diarrhea. Diarrhea, or watery stools, is a common problem of early childhood. Sometimes it is difficult to tell whether your infant is having *diarrheal stools* (which are generally caused by infections) or *more frequent loose stools* (which are usually due to diet). One way to tell is to notice whether or not the stools are formed in any way, and whether they are the same color as usual.

Diarrheal stools are watery, without any formed elements, and may be accompanied by cramps causing your baby to cry with the bowel movement. Often a baby with diarrhea will not be eating normally, will have a fever, and will be less alert. As in the case with vomiting, your baby can become dehydrated quickly if the lost fluid is not replaced. Call the doctor if you think your baby has diarrhea. As the condition is naturally worrisome, it will help you to get advice.

Eye Discharge. In the first few days, many babies have a yellowish discharge from their eyes. This is normal; it is a response to the antibiotic drops or ointment placed in their eyes after delivery. This discharge can be wiped away with a clean, wet cotton ball.

Another common cause of eye discharge in infants is a plugged tear duct. This is probably the situation if you notice increased tears or small amounts of sticky discharge in one or both eyes, particularly when the baby awakens. It results from plugging of the nasolacrimal duct, which drains excess tears from the eyes to the inside of the nose. A plugged nasolacrimal duct nearly always opens up on its own, though it may take months to do so. You can help clear it up by applying a warm washcloth and gently massaging the area over the duct.

If the baby's eyelids become increasingly red and swollen, and a thick profuse discharge develops, an infection may be present. Infections must be treated with antibiotics, given by drops to the eyes or by oral medication. They are relatively rare, however.

Fever. Fever in an infant is defined as a temperature greater than 100.4° F taken rectally or greater than 99.5° F taken orally. Often, when a baby is wrapped up too warmly, its temperature will rise. If your baby has a fever, try unwrapping him or her and retaking the temperature. If the fever persists for eight hours, any baby under two months of age should be seen by a physician and examined for signs of infection. Older babies can be treated initially with acetaminophen (Tylenol, Datril, and other brands) or by being bathed in lukewarm (not cold) water. Fever that continues for 24 hours should prompt you to call your physician for advice.

Fluoride Supplementation. Fluoride supplementation in childhood leads to better teeth throughout life. When children either drink fluoridated water or take fluoride drops, their growing teeth become stronger and more resistant to decay. Thus, teenagers and adults who received fluoride as children will have about half as many cavities (and dental bills) as children who did not receive fluoride. In areas that do not have fluoride added to the water supply, fluoride supplementation should be started shortly after birth and continue until about age 12. Ask your child's doctor about this.

Hernias. A hernia is a weakness in the muscle of the abdomen that allows an organ to push through. Hernias in the groin are called *inguinal hernias*; those in the the navel are called *umbilical hernias*. Inguinal hernias tend to get bigger if they aren't operated on. In addition, a piece of bowel can become stuck in this opening of the muscle wall, causing severe pain and requiring emergency surgery. Inguinal hernias in children should be surgically corrected. Hernias of the umbilicus are more common and much less dangerous. Most disappear in the first year and cause few complications. They rarely need any treatment.

Hiccups. Like adults, babies get hiccups when they burp or eat. Many infants had hiccups while in the uterus, and continue to have them through infancy. Harmless and painless, but sometimes annoying, hiccups can be treated by giving the baby more fluid, putting it back on the breast, or putting it over your shoulder and rubbing its back. Often a change in position helps to alleviate the problem.

Lethargy. Lethargy, or excessive sleepiness in an infant, can be an important sign of serious illness, such as infection or dehydration. A sick infant will often not want to eat, play, or look around in the usual way. A lethargic infant may sleep longer than usual and be difficult to wake up; it will not be interested in staying awake. Babies with this condition will not feed on schedule or respond to you in the usual way. If you think that your baby is behaving in this manner, call your doctor immediately.

Overfeeding. Usually not a problem with breastfed babies (since the baby determines the amount it takes), overfeeding can occur inadvertently with bottle-fed babies. Many babies just want to suck; parents interpret this need as the desire for more food. Fussy babies who require more physical comforting may be offered another bottle as a way to calm them down. If you think your newborn has eaten enough (from two to five ounces a feed) and still is hungry, give water or a pacifier. If you give formula, make sure that it is prepared correctly. Try to satisfy your baby in other ways if you feel it has eaten enough. Overfed babies often spit up more and seem uncomfortable. Remember, most physicians do not recommend solid foods before four to six months of age.

Pacifiers. Pacifiers (soothers, bickies) satisfy your infant's need to suck but are no substitute for parental attention. Although many parents object to the use of a pacifier to soothe a baby, it has saved many a parent from a sleepless night. Some hints: Use pacifiers that are made of one piece of rubber with a disk large enough so the baby cannot get the entire pacifier into its mouth and choke. Do *not* tie the pacifier to the crib or to the baby. Children have choked to death this way. Decrease the amount of time you offer it to your baby if he or she seems uninterested in it. Don't use it past six months if you can help it. There are many other ways you can satisfy an older baby.

Sleep and Wake Cycles. It is a rare infant that sleeps all night before two months. In fact, if a baby in the first few weeks of life sleeps more than five hours at a stretch, it may be ill and can become dehydrated. Most physicians suggest waking your baby after five hours and feeding it. Most babies sleep about 18 hours a day, but the intervals of sleeping and waking vary with each baby. Some babies are awake and alert for long periods of time immediately after birth and require less sleep than others. In the first days of life, sleep time prevails, with short intervals of wake time for feeding and comforting. Initially, your baby will not distinguish between day and night, but eventually will establish a diurnal rhythm. As your baby gets older, the periods of wake time increase, and the times of wakefulness at night will come at regular intervals. Gradually, your baby will sleep longer and longer at night, giving you the much-needed rest you've earned.

Sudden Infant Death Syndrome (Cribdeath). A common cause of death in the first year is a mysterious problem called sudden infant death syndrome (SIDS). Typically, an infant dies during sleep, without warning. Occasionally, a child is observed to stop breathing, gasp, or choke during sleep and is revived with mouth-to-mouth resuscitation; prevention of SIDS may thereby have occurred.

There is no known cause of this tragic occurrence. We do know that premature and frail infants are more likely to develop SIDS, and that breastfeeding may provide some protection.

As a new parent, you should realize several things about SIDS: (1) It is really quite rare, and your baby will probably not develop SIDS. (2) All parents worry about it sometimes. (3) It's common and normal to check your baby to see whether it's breathing at night. Don't be embarrassed if you feel the need to do so. It will help you sleep better. (4) The only thing we know you can do to try to prevent SIDS is to look after your baby's general physical health.

Thrush. Thrush is a mild fungus infection of the mouth caused by monilia, the same fungus that causes yeast infections in women and some diaper rashes in babies. Thrush causes white patches to form inside the infant's mouth and cheeks. These are usually not painful. Thrush must be treated with oral medication given to the baby four times a day for up to a week.

Vitamins. Doctors are currently debating whether children need vitamin supplements. If you are breastfeeding, many physicians recommend extra vitamin D. A few physicians still recommend vitamins C and A plus iron, but most breastfed infants seem to get plenty. Cow's-milk and soy-milk formulas contain the vitamins needed for normal development. Iron and other special nutrients may be needed if your baby was born prematurely. If you have questions about vitamins, ask your baby's doctor.

Vomiting. Vomiting is the forceful propulsion of the contents of a baby's stomach. It is different from spitting up, which is the regurgitation of a small amount of milk after a feed and is not serious. Vomiting, on the other hand, can occur after a feed or in no relationship to a feed. It may be caused by many problems, including infection, a blockage of the intestinal tract, and (in some cases) significant overfeeding. Infants that vomit persistently run the risk of becoming dehydrated. Because newborns do not tolerate the loss of much fluid, call your physician for advice if vomiting occurs more than once or twice in succession.

Weight Loss. Newborns lose a few ounces after delivery, but by the first week, your newborn should begin to gain weight. Most pediatricians and family physicians see new babies at two weeks of age to check for weight gain and for development. Inability to gain weight may indicate inadequate feeding, infection, or intestinal problems. If you feel your baby is losing weight, consult your physician immediately.

27 The New Mother's Physical Recovery

For the new mother, the postpartum period is also a time of physical recovery. Depending on the way your baby was delivered, and the difficulties involved, you may have to take some precautions for a while and use medication. Within a few weeks, however, most of the tender spots should be on the mend, if not already healed.

The Perineum

Torn areas and episiotomies are stitched with dissolvable suture material. These stitches heal quite quickly, usually within the first week and certainly by two or three weeks after delivery. Often, your doctor or midwife will have you sit in a shallow tub of warm water, called a sitz bath. This decreases the swelling around the labia and perineum after episiotomy. Infections are rare but occasionally occur in an area that has been stitched; you should suspect an infection if your stitches become increasingly painful two or three days after delivery.

Occasionally stitches do not heal and are quite painful without signs of infection. This usually occurs when a large number of stitches were needed. If this occurs, your health-care provider may then choose to cut some of the stitches to prevent infection and allow the skin to heal without pressure from the suture material pulling the skin. You may also be asked to have frequent sitz baths or heat-lamp treatments. The healing of the perineal area then occurs without any further stitches and usually proceeds without difficulty. If your episiotomy or laceration repair is painful or not healing well, check with your health-care provider.

Changes in the Uterus

The uterus weighs about four pounds at the time of delivery and shrinks to about three ounces within four weeks. At the time of delivery, the uterus reaches high in the abdomen, underneath the ribs. Immediately after delivery, the top of the uterus is just below the umbilicus. Within six weeks, the uterus is almost back to normal size. After delivery, the uterus contracts at irregular intervals. This process is speeded by breastfeeding, because the same hormone (oxytocin) that stimulates milk production also causes uterine contraction. As the uterus contracts, the lining or decidua is shed and passes through the vagina much like a regular period.

Hemorrhoids and Constipation

Hermorrhoids are varicose veins of the anus. They often become tender and swollen for a few days after delivery. This probably results from straining while pushing during delivery. Sitz baths, heat lamps, and medicated creams or suppositories can help relieve pain from hemorrhoids. The best medicine, however, is prevention by eating a high-fiber diet during pregnancy and making sure that you don't get constipated.

If your hemorrhoids or episiotomy stitches are painful, your first bowel movement after delivery may be quite uncomfortable. The best remedy for this situation is to keep your stool soft, and for this reason your physician or midwife may give you a stool softener during the first days after delivery. Plenty of water and a high-fiber diet will help prevent further problems with hemorrhoids. Constipation can also be a result of pain medication (particularly codeine); a stool softener can remedy this. Finally, do not resist the urge to have a bowel movement even though you are tender; holding back can also lead to constipation.

Bleeding

Bleeding after delivery varies with each woman. It is heaviest during the first 12 hours after delivery and then lessens. The amount of bleeding is estimated by doing a sanitary pad count. The average pad count in the first 24 hours is between eight and twelve pads, excluding the first few pads that were changed immediately after delivery. The pad count for the next two days averages between six and ten pads, with the last pads often being minimally stained with blood. In the first three days, blood clots or small pieces of tissue are occasionally passed. Often, blood clots come out during a contraction ("afterpain"), as the uterus decreases its size and pushes the contents out. Clots can also be passed when the woman stands or sits up after lying down. This is because blood gathers in the vagina when you lie down, and falls out when you stand up. If large clots are passed, and your sanitary pad is soaking through every 15 to 30 minutes, notify your nurse, physician, or midwife.

Blood passed during the weeks after delivery is called lochia. It gradually tapers off but can continue for as long as six weeks after delivery. Lochia is red in color in the first few days after delivery, and turns brown as time passes, finally becoming relatively clear. Sometimes brown lochia passes in relatively small amounts for a day or two, and then a surge of bright red blood with small clots occurs. This should not cause concern unless the amount of bleeding is large or cramps persist.

If your lochia continues to be heavy or increases after your discharge from the hospital, let your health-care provider know. The cause may be a small piece of tissue stuck to the wall of the uterus, preventing the uterus from fully contracting, or an infection of the uterine lining. If there is no retained tissue or sign of infection, but the lochia continues to be heavy, your physician or midwife may prescribe a drug such as Methergine or Ergotamine, which will cause the uterus to contract more forcefully and will usually reduce bleeding.

Breast Changes and Conditions

After delivery, a woman's breasts begin to ready themselves for milk production. More blood is circulated through the breast tissue, and the breasts swell, harden, and become warm. This is known as breast engorgement. The breasts first produce a watery liquid, colostrum. On about the third day after delivery, milk production begins. If the milk is not emptied from the breasts, they become tender and painful; breastfeeding will bring relief.

For women who have decided not to breastfeed, engorgement can be quite uncomfortable and less easy to remedy. Wearing a tight bra, or placing ice packs on the breasts will decrease milk production and swelling. Within a few days, your breast fullness and tenderness will subside. If necessary, your doctor can also prescribe medication to stop milk production.

Bruising around the nipples is common in breastfeeding mothers. This happens when the baby is allowed to suck on the nipples for long periods of time or fails to take the nipple and areola into the mouth while nursing. The bruising disappears in a day or two and can be prevented by making sure the baby attaches to the breast in the proper fashion (see page 192).

In the first week of breastfeeding, your nipples may become chapped. Quite painful, chapped nipples can be treated with breast cream. Using a cream such as lanolin from the beginning helps prevent this chapping. The cream should be wiped off before the baby's feeds. Keep the cracked area clean and dry to prevent infection.

Abdominal and Pelvic Floor Muscles

Through the nine months of pregnancy, your abdominal muscles have been stretched. Even after delivery, most mothers still look pregnant, partly because the abdominal muscles remain out of shape. If you have had no complications, you can begin to tone up your abdominal muscles almost immediately. Your health-care provider or exercise teacher can suggest specific exercises to tighten the abdominal muscles, as well as outline a time schedule for reconditioning your body. Check with your doctor for the go-ahead. Remember that it took many months to change your shape, and it will probably take nearly as long to return to the desired state.

The Kegel exercises you did to condition your pelvic floor muscles can now be used to regain the muscle tone you had before pregnancy. These exercises can begin a few hours after delivery without disturbing the stitches of an episiotomy. Contracting the muscles brings the tissue closer together and will aid healing. As the perineum heals and becomes less swollen, increase the length of time for your Kegel exercises. Restoring these muscle groups will prevent leakage of urine in later years and improve your sexual response.

Anemia

Anemia after delivery results from insufficient nutrition during pregnancy, or from excess blood loss during the delivery. If you were anemic before delivery, you probably will have taken iron pills or injections. Anemia from excessive blood loss is also treated with iron. Women who are anemic feel more fatigued and their bodies heal more slowly. In severe anemia, blood transfusions can replace lost blood cells rapidly, allowing you to quickly regain your strength.

Leg Cramps and Ankle Swelling

Many women complain of leg cramps and ankle swelling after delivery. Both are common occurrences in pregnancy and usually disappear within two weeks of delivery. Leg cramps may be a result of a mineral imbalance, or may just reflect muscle spasm. You can prevent cramping by wearing support stockings and making sure your diet is high in calcium, phosphorus, and vitamin D. In rare instances, cramps or pain in the legs may reflect blood clots. In these cases, one leg becomes quite painful, swollen, and warm to the touch. If you notice these symptoms, call your physician immediately.

In women with varicose veins, ankle swelling may take longer to clear up. The swelling is caused by excess fluid in the body and often occurs with preeclampsia. Wearing support stockings and exercising the legs can increase circulation and decrease swelling. Walking as much as possible helps to increase the circulation in your legs.

Diet and Weight Loss in Breast- and Bottle-feeding Mothers

Within a few days after delivery, a woman loses two or three pounds of fluid, about two pounds from the shrinking of the uterus, and several pounds from the baby and the amniotic fluid. Even after this weight loss, most women weigh more than they did before they were pregnant. The remaining weight is stored as fat; you can lose it by proper dieting and exercise.

Many women lose the remaining pounds slowly by watching their calories and getting regular exercise. To prevent obesity, you should try to get back to your normal weight after delivery. The caloric requirements for a nonbreastfeeding mother are between 1,500 and 2,000 calories per day. A breastfeeding mother requires more calories, about 2,000 to 2,300 calories per day, including plenty of protein. You do not have to drink milk to produce it, but it is important to get enough calcium and to drink plenty of fluids.

The postpartum period is not a good time to go on a crash diet. New mothers need a lot of energy, and losing more than one-and-a-half pounds per week may increase fatigue. A regular exercise program and a well-balanced diet are the keys to normal weight loss. Ask your health-care provider for information about your ideal weight and the best diet for you.

Recovery after Caesarean Section

The postpartum course for the caesarean mother varies. The surgical incision is about six inches long. It is usually located parallel to, but below, where the elastic strip on bikini underpants goes across the abdomen. Most incisions are closed with clips that are removed after 72 hours. The incision is then held together by adhesive strips (steri-strips), which remain in place until they fall off. Most caesarean mothers experience a burning or pulling sensation from their stitches for about a week. The incision and the skin below it can feel numb or tingle for six weeks or longer.

The surgical scar is quite painful for a day or two, and most women need pain medication during the first 24 hours. As the pain lessens, you can receive further medication, but you have to ask for it. The medication is usually codeine or a similar drug. It does not interfere with breastfeeding and is safe for the new baby. Constipation is a usual side effect of such drugs; be sure to ask for a laxative if it has not already been ordered. The other severe pain after caesarean section comes from gas that results from the interruption of normal digestion because of surgery. These gas pains can be sharp but will disappear quickly. They can sometimes be lessened by drinking an antacid/antiflatulent liquid.

You may need to use a bedpan until you feel able to get out of bed, usually 12 to 24 hours after delivery. Because a catheter was placed in the urethra during surgery, urinating may be uncomfortable the first few times. Bowel movements can be quite painful if you are constipated and have to bear down using the muscles that have been cut. A laxative and stool softener, as well as high-fiber foods, will help ease the pain. Even though it hurts, moving around and walking as soon as possible will make the pain go away faster and promote healing.

An intravenous line usually remains in your arm for about 24 hours after surgery. It will be removed as soon as you can drink liquids, unless you need intravenous medication. If the i.v. site is painful or swollen, ask for a hot compress. Blood is usually taken once after delivery to be sure you didn't lose too much blood. Most women are discharged after a four-day stay in the hospital and are seen two weeks later for a check-up.

Recovery from a caesarean section is much like recovery from any surgical procedure. The first day or two after surgery, you will feel tired and be quite aware of the incision. Moving, bending, and walking will seem very difficult. The incision is usually well closed in one week, and six weeks after surgery the tissue is mended. It often takes up to six months for the scar to fade. Most women are out of bed a few days after surgery, performing all of the activities new mothers need to do. Nursing can proceed in a regular fashion after caesarean section and is encouraged. But fatigue lasts longer than after vaginal delivery, often for several weeks. Extra rest is the best treatment for this fatigue; it will help your body heal.

There used to be a rule in obstetrics that "once a section, always a section." In the past five years, however, many obstetricians have offered women a *trial of labor*. This means that a woman who has previously had a caesarean section may labor normally, although usually with a uterine-contraction monitor on. If all goes well, the delivery is done vaginally. This a well-accepted option now. If you want more information on a trial of labor, ask your physician or midwife about this option.

28 Renewing Your Sexual Relationship

At about six weeks, you should be checked by your physician or midwife. By this time, your body will be mostly back to normal. (Your weight and muscle tone will take more time.) Your family will have settled into a routine, and you and your partner may have already resumed intercourse. Your health-care provider will ask about your physical and emotional health and answer any questions you have. He or she will want to know whether you are having problems with your breasts, whether your stitches have healed, and whether you have had a period yet. Then, a physical exam will be performed, much like the one you had when you first went to your health-care provider for prenatal care. He or she will take your blood pressure, check your weight and urine, examine your breasts and abdominal muscles, and perform a pelvic exam to determine the shape and condition of your cervix, uterus, and ovaries. The vagina will be examined to check for looseness or tightness, and to see that all stitches or lacerations have healed. Your health-care provider should then discuss methods of contraception with you if this was not already done after delivery.

Many women prefer not to have intercourse until the postpartum exam has been completed, but this is not necessary. Usually by two weeks after delivery, lochia is scant, stitches are well healed, and the swelling and pain in the perineum has subsided. Comfort is the limiting factor for most couples. If you have a lot of pain when you first try intercourse, try again in a week or so, making sure you are well lubricated. Most health-care providers will offer information about intercourse and will answer any questions you have about resuming sexual activity. Feel free to ask any questions about intercourse, pain, bleeding, or anything else that is of concern.

Contraception

It is rare to ovulate earlier than four weeks after delivery. The average nonbreastfeeding mother first ovulates at three months. Breastfeeding mothers ovulate five months after delivery on the average, but this is quite variable. Thus, *any* mother can get pregnant within a few months after delivery, and contraception should be used as soon as you begin having intercourse. Talk your situation over with your health-care provider.

Here are your main choices among methods of contraception:

● **Oral contraceptives (birth control pills)** are very effective. They can interfere with your milk production and thus are usually not recommended if you are breastfeeding. Mothers who bottle-feed can begin the pill soon after delivery.

● **Diaphragms with spermicide** are quite effective if used every time you have intercourse. They provide good methods of birth control for breastfeeding women. Because the vagina often is shaped differently after delivery, your old diaphragm will need to be refitted. For every ten pounds you lose, your diaphragm size should be checked to prevent slippage during intercourse, which could lead to an unwanted pregnancy.

● **Other barrier methods** include foam and condoms, vaginal suppositories and condoms, or condoms alone. Their effectiveness is good if used correctly and in combination.

● **An intrauterine device (IUD)** is also very effective, and can be fitted at the six-week exam.

● **Sterilization** is a choice for couples who feel they have enough children after the most recent birth.

● **Tubal ligation**, which involves cutting and tying, clipping, or burning the fallopian tubes, can be performed immediately after delivery or at a later time. Some states require that the consent form for tubal ligation be signed six weeks before delivery.

● **Vasectomy** is a procedure for the man that is comparable to tubal ligation; it can be performed at any time and becomes effective within a couple of months after the procedure. Neither procedure interferes with sexual performance. They are generally not reversible.

Resuming Lovemaking

The reestablishment of a sexual relationship after delivery can be a source of anxiety for many new parents. While a man is often quite anxious to resume lovemaking, his partner may be very fatigued, sore from an episiotomy and feeling very little desire to do much more than sleep and care for the baby. She may find it hard to think of herself as romantic when she is overweight, has stretch marks on her abdomen and breasts, and feels like a baby-feeding machine. This difference in desire for sex often pushes partners apart at a time when new parents need to relate to each other as well as to the new baby.

Even if intercourse is deferred until the mother is more physically recovered, it is important for a couple to resume some kind of sexual contact as soon as possible. What seems to be a common and important need for most couples is physical closeness, and a few tender moments of holding and kissing. Many couples find that the arrival of a new baby is a time to experiment with sex, to discover new ways of giving pleasure and showing affection. The hardest thing, it seems, is finding enough uninterrupted time. Being creative and going slowly can make the return to intercourse enjoyable and painless.

Most physicians recommend no intercourse for between two to six weeks after delivery, to prevent infection and promote healing. There are many things that a couple can do to rekindle their intimate relationship without intercourse. Hugging, kissing, manual manipulation of the penis or clitoris, and oral-genital sex are permitted. The use of a vibrator to help the woman achieve orgasm is acceptable, as long as it is not placed inside the vagina. Neither partner needs to feel guilty about giving the other pleasure by manual stimulation.

After childbirth, many women feel that it takes longer to reach orgasm than before. This delay in arousal is often related to changing hormone levels and fatigue. Setting aside time for prolonged foreplay and experimenting with new patterns of lovemaking can help you adjust to this change.

Many couples resume sexual intercourse before the recommended abstinence period is up. Unless there is heavy bleeding or infection, there is little danger of doing physical damage to the woman's healing body.

Many women experience pain with intercourse, especially after an episiotomy. Even mild pressure on the vaginal floor with a finger can be a painful experience for weeks after delivery. By avoiding the pressure of the penis against the back part of the vagina and redirecting it to the clitoral area, pain during insertion can be minimized. Thrusting should be limited during the first lovemaking sessions, and a woman should direct the entry of the penis into the vagina to determine the most favorable angle. The missionary position can be quite painful for the woman. As in pregnancy, other positions, such as the side-to-side (face-to-face) or the woman on top may be more comfortable. Lovemaking after delivery feels different than it did before pregnancy because the woman's body experiences real anatomical changes that affect the mechanics of sex as well as the sensation.

In many women, especially those who are breastfeeding, vaginal lubrication can be a problem. The vagina, which was usually quite wet during pregnancy, is now dry. Prolonged foreplay and the use of a vaginal lubricant, contraceptive cream, or oil to ease entry of the penis into the vagina can help.

The breasts of a lactating woman are often tender, and nipple stimulation will cause them to leak. When stimulated, lactating breasts will spurt milk. Many men feel uncomfortable with leaking breasts and feel embarrassed if they happen to get a taste of milk during lovemaking. Some men feel confused and conflicted over their partner's dual roles of wife and mother. Breasts that once were objects of sexual stimulation are now the objects of milk production, and often both partners feel that their sexual interaction is interrupted by this normal physiologic change. Women often notice that their nipples are not as responsive to sexual stimulation as they once were. This lack of response usually returns when breastfeeding is discontinued. Some women find that they become sexually aroused during breastfeeding. This is a common, normal response.

Here are some suggestions that may help you achieve a renewed intimacy. Set aside time for lovemaking after your baby has been fed. Knowing that her baby is asleep and content can help a mother relax and concentrate on her and her partner's satisfaction. Also, the nipples tend to be less sensitive after a feed. So that you won't be disturbed by baby noises, place the baby in an adjoining room. Find new areas to caress and stimulate each other, avoiding tender or healing areas, or parts of the body that make one or both partners uncomfortable. For many couples, massage of the back, neck, upper arms, inner thighs, and knees can be very satisfying. Finding comfortable positions that avoid pressure on full breasts or a tender abdomen will make both partners respond more easily. Prolonged foreplay and the use of extra lubricant can prevent a lot of discomfort.

The need for private time, alone or with your partner, is perhaps the most important key to resuming a healthy sexual relationship. Both parents focus so much attention on a new infant, or other children after the birth of a new sibling, that often they have little time for themselves. While long mornings in bed together with coffee and the Sunday newspapers may not be an option, twenty minutes for a hot bath, taking a walk, or going out for coffee or a drink can provide relaxation and reduce tension. Couples who are able to take a night or weekend away when they feel comfortable enough to leave their baby, and have time for uninterrupted sleep, lovemaking, and time alone together, find that their sexual relationship has been renewed and recharged. Remember that a visiting parent or friend in the next room can often inhibit your lovemaking. Getting out for a few hours, or leaving your infant with an experienced friend or relative can be the best aphrodisiac.

If you find you are having a lot of trouble reestablishing your sexual relationship, ask your health-care provider for advice. He or she may recommend that you both come in for counseling, or may refer you to a specialist if necessary.

29 Emotional Changes after Pregnancy and Delivery

Many people view pregnancy, delivery, and childrearing as the most important events of their lives. Every parent has expectations of how this experience should be. Television has also led us to believe that this experience can be perfect from start to finish: babies quietly sleeping in beautifully decorated rooms, mothers and fathers rested and raving about how wonderful it is to be the parents of a perfect baby. Almost all parents will tell you that the actual experience differed greatly from the anticipated one. Even those who have experienced childbirth before will tell you that every birth is different, that every child is different, and that their feelings about each childbirth experience and outcome are different.

Changes in Lifestyle

When you make the decision to have a child you choose to alter your lifestyle and life experiences. You cannot entirely predict, however, how your life will actually change. You shouldn't be surprised, therefore, if being a parent is different from your expectations. Your infant's needs, the amount of fatigue you experience, and changes in your feelings about your job, your mate, or your priorities in life may affect your whole outlook. Day by day, you will learn new skills—how to recognize your child's needs, as well as your own need for sleep and privacy—and you will figure out how to cope or whom to ask for help.

Most babies take some time to develop a schedule, but some fit into household routines very quickly. Some babies are quiet from birth, while others are noisy and active. No parent gets used to a colicky, fussy baby that cries for hours each day, but parents learn to cope with nearly any problem.

Don't expect to have all the answers or feel comfortable with all the changes at once. Read about what you might expect, and ask lots of questions when you talk with your health-care provider, your friends with children, or whoever you think can offer helpful advice. Give yourself and your family time to adjust to one another. Here are some guidelines for coping, as suggested by experts on early childhood:

- The responsibilities of parenthood are learned; do what you can to get informed.
- Obtain help from your partner, dependable friends, relatives, and neighbors. Don't be afraid to ask for help.
- Make friends with people who have children.
- Don't overload yourself with unimportant tasks.
- Don't move shortly before or soon after the baby arrives.
- Don't be overconcerned with keeping up appearances.
- Get plenty of rest and sleep. Take naps when your baby sleeps.
- Don't be a nurse to friends and relatives during this period.
- Confer and consult with your partner, family, and experienced friends and relatives. Discuss your fears and worries.
- Don't give up outside interests, but cut down on outside responsibilities, rearrange schedules, and do less.
- Arrange for babysitters and daycare early.
- Get a family doctor or pediatrician early.*

Baby Blues and Postpartum Depression

In the first days and weeks after childbirth, 70 to 80 percent of all women experience to some degree the emotional changes that are traditionally called the "baby blues." They are caused by a combination of fatigue, anxiety, and changes in hormone levels. Many women feel sad and weepy, some get very worried about their lack of maternal feelings, and others feel anxious and scared that they will not be able to handle the responsibility of parenthood. It is common to have difficulty sleeping and concentrating. "Baby blues" usually begin within the first four days after delivery and can go on for a week or two. They often occur at about the same

*List adapted from R. E. Gordon, E. E. Kapostins, and K. K. Gordon, "Factors in Postpartum Emotional Adjustment," *Obstetrics and Gynecology* 25 (1965): 158–66.

time your breasts become swollen and tender. In some women these feelings are delayed a week or so.

All of these feelings are normal. Although sometimes intense and alarming, they are temporary and will soon fade. Lack of sleep makes these negative feelings worse, and increasing your sleep can lessen their intensity. Remind yourself that the "blues" will pass; seek support from your family and friends. Occasionally feelings of depression or inadequacy last longer than a week or two and increase in intensity; professional counseling and possibly medication may then be necessary.

Usually "baby blues" fade quickly, and with a night's rest, feelings of inadequacy go away. If they do not fade, however, the new mother may begin to feel completely inadequate and helpless, overcome by her responsibilities to her infant or family, unable to do anything to interrupt these feelings. This situation, called *postpartum depression*, is more serious. It can occur in women with good support systems, with concerned, helpful partners. It requires professional evaluation and treatment by a psychiatrist or psychologist.

There are as many causes for postpartum depression as there are women who experience it. Many women suffer from depressive symptoms but cannot identify them, and wait months before seeking help. Here are some of the signs of a postpartum depression:

loss of appetite	**rejecting the baby**
confused thoughts	**thinking the baby is dead**
bad dreams	**confusing day and night**
excessive crying	**feeling trapped**
excessive sweating	**forgetfulness**
feeling inferior	**feeling physically violent**
mind going blank	**suicidal thoughts**
increased alcohol intake	**excessive guilt or anxiety**
hopeless feelings	**refusing to feed the baby**
insomnia	**lack of interest in life****

Having one or two of the symptoms listed above does not necessarily mean you are experiencing a postpartum depression. However, it is important to recognize the signs and symptoms early and to ask for help. Many women feel ashamed of such feelings and put off talking about their symptoms of depression, which makes them feel more guilty and depressed because they cannot cope with the situation. Often, the woman's partner recognizes the

**List adapted from Judith Gansberg and Arthur Mostel, *The Second Nine Months* (New York: Tribeca Communications, 1984), p. 160.

symptoms and calls the doctor for help. If you are feeling depressed and have any of the symptoms listed above, seek professional help as soon as possible.

Is the World Passing Me By?

Many new parents, especially mothers who are often at home for most of the day and out of contact with the working world, feel that in the process of becoming a parent, and focusing on the new infant's needs 24 hours a day, that they have or will become boring. The intense concentration required to take care of a new baby, coupled with the inability to do much of anything else in the two months following delivery, leaves most parents exhausted. They don't read newspapers and magazines, they don't answer letters, and their conversation is full of talk about feeding schedules and diaper services. Many women feel that their intellectual functioning has decreased and they are doomed to talk about diarrhea and colic forever. Take heart! You are not boring, but appropriately focused on your infant. This focus on your baby is necessary and is a sign of healthy bonding. As you become more comfortable with your baby, and the baby gets on a regular schedule, you will find more time to get involved with those activities you have put on hold.

Jealousy and Anger

Jealousy is commonly felt during the postpartum period by mothers, fathers and children, friends and relatives. Fathers often feel jealous of the new baby, to whom the mother devotes the bulk of her time. Many men miss the attention from their partners and the uninterrupted intimate contact.

A new mother often feels jealous when the attention that was focused on her during pregnancy turns entirely to the new baby. Presents, visitors, and phone calls all revolve around the new baby. A mother may feel angry at the loss of autonomy and the need to focus all of her attention and time on the baby. Expressing these feelings to your partner, friends, or physician can lessen their intensity. Often, time alone will ease these feelings.

Anger is an emotional signal that tells you that you are not getting what you want. It is difficult to accept that one feels anger, especially toward a new baby, one's partner, or one's family, at a time that should be so full of love and joy. However, new parents often feel angry about the changes in their lifestyle as the result of the birth of their child. Working parents who are now at home often miss the excitement of the job and feel angry at the loss of independence and free time. If the birth of the baby resulted from an unplanned pregnancy, both parents can feel angry at each other or at the baby for disrupting their regular routines. If the birth of the baby leads to more attention from parents or in-laws with whom you don't get along well, conflict can result.

A good way to resolve the angry feelings is to figure out what it is that you are not getting—be it sleep, sex, time alone, or help with the chores—and to find a way to get it. This requires facing the fact that you are angry, talking about it, and finding solutions or compromises. Sometimes it takes a while for some of the issues to be resolved, but talking about what makes you angry is the only way to alleviate frustration and tension.

It is not unusual for parents to feel anger toward a crying child, frustration at a baby that will not go to sleep, or despair when they need rest and sleep. Most parents are able to identify these feelings and ask for help from their partners, family members, or friends. However, some parents, who feel overwhelmed and disturbed, translate these feelings of anger into physical violence. If you find yourself shaking, hitting, or feeling that you want to harm your child, call your physician, minister, or a parents' hotline for help and advice. Physical outbursts are signals to parents that they need professional help.

If you find yourself unable to cope with your home situation or child, you can call Parents Anonymous: 1-800-421-0353. At Parents Anonymous, someone is always on hand to give you advice or help. You will not have to give your name or provide details if you do not wish to do so.

A Feeling of Fulfillment

The first few weeks of parenting tend to be exhausting, demanding, and emotionally stressful. In spite of the difficulties, the vast majority of parents regard the experience as a positive one.

Why is this so? Part of it has to do with the joy of holding, nurturing, and being with a new person. Babies are very attractive and responsive, and they are easy to love. Another factor is the feeling of working together that a couple often develops. The demands of caring for a child can draw a couple closer, through sharing the work of parenting. Finally, there is a feeling of doing something you really believe in and care about. Most likely you chose to become parents, and the care of your child is a fulfillment of this wish.

RECOMMENDED RESOURCES

Brewer, Gail Sforza. *The Pregnancy After 30 Workbook*. Emmaus, Pennsylvania: Rodale Press, 1978. A lovely book for the older new mother written by a well-respected American childbirth expert.

Gansberg, Judith, and Arthur Mostel. *The Second Nine Months*. New York: Tribeca Communications, 1984. A comprehensive look at the emotional and sexual changes women go through during the months after delivery. Frank and informative.

30 After the First Four Weeks

When the baby has been home for a month or so, practical decisions have to be made about establishing a daily routine. Will the mother go back to work? What sort of care should the baby have if both parents are working? The first four weeks have been a time of adjustment; now is the time for settling into family life, balancing your needs as an adult with the needs of the growing child.

Going Back to Work

The decision to return to work is a difficult one for a new mother. Some women must return to work in order to stay afloat financially. Others choose to go back to work. In either case, most working mothers feel some guilt about leaving their babies and wonder whether they are harming their children. They must depend on babysitters or daycare centers, and worry constantly about the care and attention their children receive from strangers.

Going back to work complicates a daily schedule. For full-time workers, the schedule can be grueling. Getting up early, feeding the baby and perhaps other children, dropping the baby off at daycare, and getting yourself to work is a superhuman task. To survive the daily routine, you'll need to limit the amount of housework that gets done on any one day or weekend and delegate household chores to your partner or other children. Receiving support from your partner in the form of help with chores or shopping makes life tolerable.

Having a supportive partner helps the working mother cope with the stress of a work schedule and with ambivalence about being separated from her child. A father who willingly shares in childcare and actively wants to be involved in childrearing can be most helpful to a woman who is returning to work. If the mother's partner does not support her decision to return to work, however, problems can arise quickly. Often the working mother feels torn between her partner's needs and her own. Some men resent the extra chores they are asked to do, and this becomes a source of conflict and stress. If you talk about the issues related to returning to work before making the decision, you can reduce tension and conflict.

No matter how good your daycare situation is, returning to work is traumatic. The first few times you leave your new infant can be painful emotional experiences. Many women feel depressed until they arrive at work and get into their work routine. For a child, the most difficult time to enter daycare is between about eight and eighteen months of age when "stranger anxiety" is highest. For this reason, many experts recommend that mothers return to work either before or after this critical period.

On the positive side, many women feel a great emotional boost from returning to work. The opportunity to be with adults, to be recognized for their abilities by coworkers, and to get a break from parenting provides needed satisfaction and variety for many women. Often, they find new enthusiasm for being with their children once parenting is no longer a 24-hour activity. In addition, surrogate childcare is not harmful, as long as attention and love are provided. In fact, recent studies have shown that children in babysitting environments learn to socialize more easily with other children and adapt to school more easily than children who had stayed at home full-time.

Thus, while it is natural to feel some discomfort about leaving a child in someone else's care, working does not make you a bad parent. Mothers who work must make an extra effort to have quality time with their children, but they enjoy the time they spend with their children immensely.

Some hints for the working mother are as follows:

- Have your child's clothing and food ready if you have out-of-home daycare. Keep all of the baby paraphernalia in one bag in a regular place.
- Stagger your schedule with your partner so you each have time alone with your child, as well as some time to yourselves.
- Take time to play with your child when you get home.
- If you work far from home, consider placing your child in a daycare center close to your job. You can then spend time in the car with your child as you commute.

• Plan to cook on the weekends, and freeze food in portions. Then, when you come home from work, you can spend your time with your child, not in the kitchen.

• Consider hiring a babysitter on Saturday so you can do your errands quickly.

• Always leave emergency phone numbers with your caregiver, and let people at work know where you are in case an emergency call comes in for you.

• Try to have some back-up childcare available (such as a babysitting co-op) in case your regular caregiver becomes ill.

• Divide up the childcare duties to be performed with your partner. This may prevent disagreements or resentment in regard to parenting issues.*

Daycare Options

As Brooke McKamy Beebe says in her *Tips for Toddlers*, finding an appropriate daycare situation is vital to the well-being of every parent. You don't have to be working in order to use daycare. To keep your spirits up, it is important that you be able to leave your child for an afternoon and get out alone or with friends. The choice of who will take care of your child and where the daycare will take place is often a difficult one. Some women prefer to have a relative take care of their babies, while others feel that having a trustworthy outsider be the caregiver is a better arrangement for all concerned. Having a relative provide care often assures the parents that the child will be well looked after, but it is often difficult to ask a relative to vacuum or do the laundry. For those who do not have a family member close by who is willing to do daycare, there are many options: daycare centers, homecare, and babysitting cooperatives.

To be licensed by the state, daycare centers must fulfill certain requirements regarding the provision of care to children. Most states have a maximum child-to-caregiver ratio, as well as standards for facilities, emergency procedures, food served, and the level of care or education provided to each child. If you are considering a daycare center, call your state's Department of Social Services to check on the requirements for licensing and any information or complaints the state has received about the centers you are considering. Investigate the situation at each daycare center you are considering, and ask what the qualifications of the staff are. Visit the daycare center and observe the children who are there. Do they look happy? Do you think they are receiving the proper

*List adapted from Brooke McKamy Beebe, *Tips for Toddlers* (New York: Dell Publishing Company, 1983), pp. 133–44.

amount of attention? Are there enough toys to go around? Is the facility in good condition? Ask how they deal with a sick child, and find out how the center handles accidents and injuries. It also is a good idea to ask the same questions of parents with children who attend the daycare center and to talk with them about their impressions of the facility. Once you decide on a center, stay in close contact with the staff. Occasionally drop in unannounced to check on the care your child is being given.

For very young children, someone who keeps a few children in her home is often preferable to a large daycare center. If you are considering this kind of care, there are many places to look for a person who sits for children in her home or is willing to come into yours. Advertisements in the local paper, in a church bulletin, or on the supermarket bulletin board are good sources of information. Inquiring at the local senior citizen's center or at the department of employment can often give you leads on babysitters or housekeepers. Be sure to let your friends and relatives know that you are looking for a home-care situation. Often word of mouth is the best way to find a good babysitter.

Screen the candidates over the phone first, and ask for references. If your phone conversation seems promising, arrange an interview at the place where the care will be provided. Examine the home and determine whether the set-up will provide the desired amount of love, safety, and stimulation for your child. If your child will be transported, make sure a car seat is available for your child's use. Find out whether the caregiver is in good health and has a backup person in case he or she becomes ill. Perhaps the most important thing to determine is whether the caregiver's philosophy of childrearing is compatible with yours. As with the daycare center, determine the emergency protocol for injuries, accidents, and illnesses.

If you are fortunate to have a caregiver who comes to your home, you can tailor your requests for childcare to your specific wishes. If you can afford a housekeeper to watch your child while she cleans the house, your life will be much improved. Before hiring a caregiver, interview each applicant carefully and check out the individual's references carefully. Make sure that the person you hire is in good health and trustworthy.

Another option for parents of young children is a babysitting cooperative. Generally, cooperatives are made up of the parents of four or five children who agree to spend one day a week babysitting all of the children in their homes. Since the parents themselves are the babysitters, the cost is minimal and you can assure yourself of the care your child will be receiving. This situation is often ideal for parents who work part-time or not at all. A babysitting cooperative can also help in the evening, if members of the cooperative trade babysitting nights. It is often good to have the co-op to fall back on in case you need an evening away on the spur of the moment.

A Preview of Your Baby's Development

Your baby will grow day by day. One of the most exciting things for you as parents will be to observe these daily changes and to enjoy each task your baby masters on the way to becoming an independent person. This excitement does not stop when your baby begins to walk but continues throughout the years you and your child are together The rate of development and growth is different

Developmental Milestones in the First Six Months*

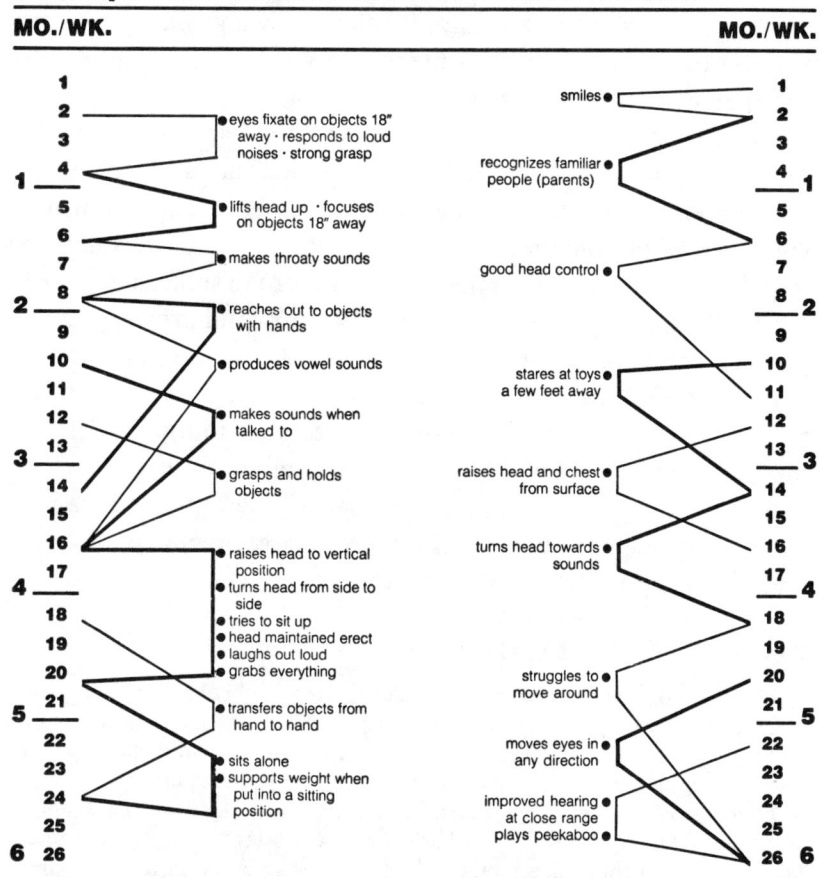

*Adapted from the Denver Developmental Screening Test.

for each child, even within the same family. It depends on inherited factors and environmental opportunities. Your child will develop skills at different rates. Thus, it is not uncommon for a child to be an early walker, but slow in talking. If you are worried about your child's development, discuss this with your doctor.

The chart on page 235 outlines some of the developmental milestones that are usually seen during the first six months of life. The time frame shown for each milestone reflects the average age at which babies can perform certain tasks, as determined by developmental experts. Because children vary so much, this chart cannot predict when your child will reach a specific milestone.

The Experience of Parenthood

Most parents find the experience of having children to be different than they imagined. Some are surprised by the time and energy parenting requires. Others find themselves unexpectedly anxious and uncertain. Many are overwhelmed by the intense love, attachment, and fascination they have for their growing child. For nearly all, the experience is more intense, more emotional, and more fulfilling than they had thought.

Thus, in spite of the pain, the anxiety, the hard work, and the sacrifices, you will probably be glad you became a parent. Of all life's experiences, there's something very special about raising a child—helping your new daughter or son make those small but important strides toward understanding a broad smile, a discovery, a new food, a new skill, and so on. As your child grows, you find yourself growing too, in experiences, memories, and maturity.

In this book, the authors have tried to let you know what to expect about pregnancy and the time immediately following delivery, as well as to prepare you for the unpredictable. We urge new parents to make use of the resources available, to ask questions, and to become active participants in the experience of pregnancy, delivery, and childrearing. Now it is up to you!

RECOMMENDED RESOURCES

Beebe, Brooke McKamy. *Tips for Toddlers*. New York: Dell Publishing Company, 1983. A book of lists on how to handle a toddler, with good suggestions for daycare options. This book is the companion to *Best Bets for Babies*, another book of helpful hints for new parents written by the same author.

Fraiberg, Selma. *The Magic Years: Understanding and Handling the Problems of Early Childhood*. New York: Charles Scribner's Sons, 1959. An outstanding book about your child's development through the years and your role as a parent.

Checklists and Worksheets

A. THINGS TO DO BEFORE GETTING PREGNANT

Step 1: Review the Risks of Pregnancy for You

☐ Review your medical status and any medications you are on.

☐ Obtain genetic counseling, if indicated.

☐ Review risks to health in your environment, home, and workplace.

Step 2: Get Yourself in the Best Shape Possible

☐ Find out whether you are immune to rubella. If not, get a rubella shot three months before trying to get pregnant.

☐ If you are overweight, lose weight.

☐ Build up your physical fitness.

☐ Limit or stop alcohol and smoking.

☐ Be sure you are on a balanced, nutritious diet. If you are a vegetarian, make sure you have adequate zinc and B_{12} intake.

☐ Begin taking a prenatal vitamin or folic acid supplement.

☐ Choose the right partner!

Step 3: Make a Decision to Try to Get Pregnant

☐ Stop your contraception.

☐ Begin recording the day each menstrual period begins, to make it easier to determine when you get pregnant.

☐ Find a health-care provider who suits your needs. If you have any questions or concerns, see that person before you get pregnant.

B. FERTILITY CHART

Name: _____

Age: _____

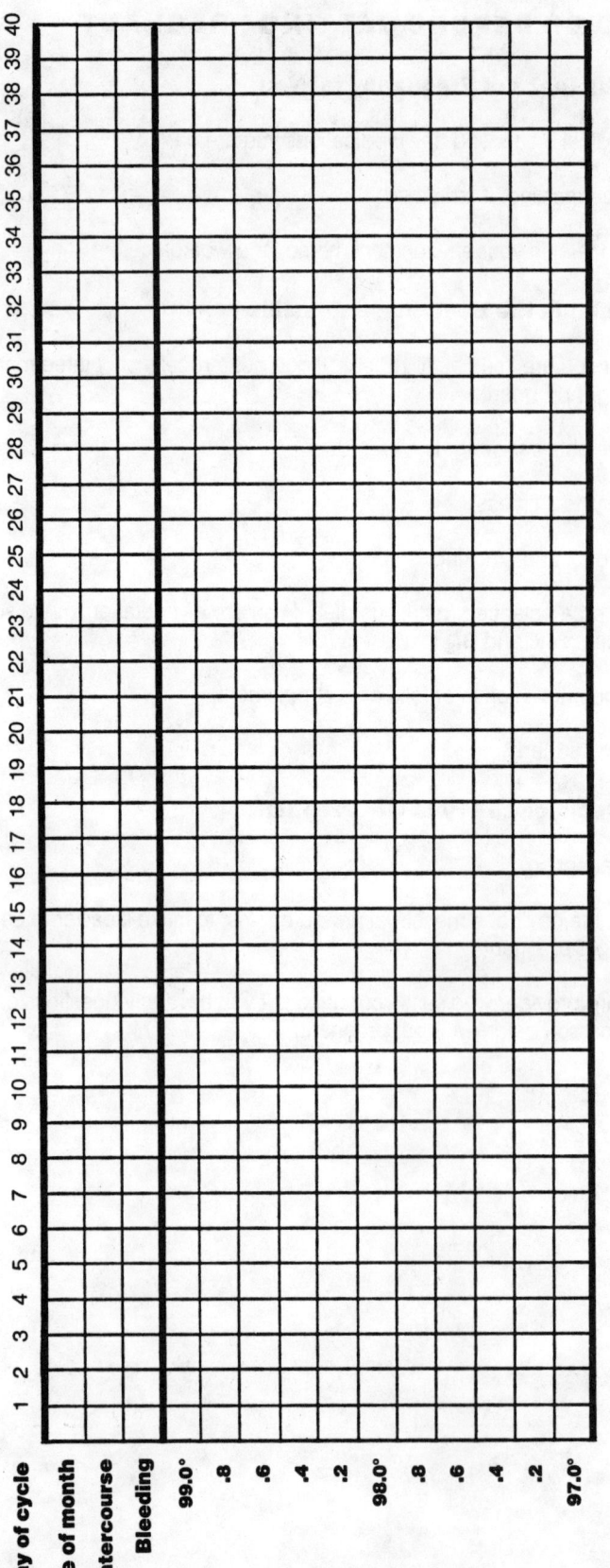

Use these symbols:

*for intercourse

For bleeding
S   for spotting
M for moderate flow (up to 4 pads or tampons per day)
H for heavy flow (5 or more pads or tampons per day)

C. WHAT TO LOOK FOR IN A HEALTH-CARE PROVIDER

Name of health-care provider _____

Address _____

Phone _____

1. Attitude and philosophy

☐ childbirth classes?

☐ participation of partner in whole childbirth process?

☐ participation of children?

☐ technological interventions?

☐ who makes final decisions?

☐ patient education?

☐ birthing positions?

☐ informed consent for procedures?

☐ anesthesia?

☐ episiotomy?

☐ caesarean section?

2. Facilities

☐ staff?

☐ hours available for appointments?

☐ after-hours calls?

☐ parking?

☐ waiting time for appointments?

☐ back-up if provider is out of town?

3. Where does birth take place?

☐ hospital affiliations?

☐ home-style birth room in hospital?

☐ home birthing center outside hospital?

☐ in your own home?

4. Fees

☐ insurance coverage?

☐ when are payments due?

☐ extra fees for procedures such as caesarean section, twins?

☐ are fees prorated?

5. Referrals

☐ to whom?

☐ under what circumstances?

6. Other questions

☐ _____

☐ _____

☐ _____

☐ _____

☐ _____

☐ _____

D. YOUR OWN LABORATORY TEST CHECKLIST

Blood type (circle one)   A   B   AB   O

Rh (circle one)   +   −

                                    date   reading

Hematocrit   _____   _____

                                    _____   _____

                                    _____   _____

Rubella titer (circle one)   +   −

Syphilis blood test (circle one)   +   −

Pap test (circle one)   normal   abnormal

                                    date   reading

Urine Culture   _____   _____

                                    _____   _____

Alpha fetal protein (circle one)   **normal**   **abnormal**

E. RISK ASSESSMENT WORKSHEET

By showing you a scoring system for estimating risk at mid-pregnancy and when labor begins, we will give you an idea of how health-care providers routinely assess the chance of complications in pregnancy. As you work out a score for yourself, you should gain a sense of whether you and your baby are at high or low risk for difficulty.

Your score is by no means a sure estimate of possible problems. Complications do occur in low-risk women, although less often than in those who are at high risk. Thus, what you learn from this work-

sheet can only provide you with a rough estimate of your risk. You should discuss any concerns or questions about your chance of complications with your health-care provider.

There are a number of scoring systems available. We will use a modification of one that was developed for doctors a few years ago in Minnesota (Edwards et al., "A Simplified Antepartum Risk-Scoring System", *Obstetrics and Gynecology* 54 [1979]: 237–40).

Risk Assessment at Mid-Pregnancy

For each question that you answer with *yes*, circle the number in the right-hand column.

Questions about previous pregnancies   Points

Have you ever had a miscarriage or therapeutic abortion?	1
More than one?	2
Have you had five or more children?	2
Have you ever had a child that was stillborn or died within one week of birth?	5
More than one?	7
Have you ever had a caesarean section?	5
Have you ever given birth to a child with a major deformity?	1
Did you have preeclampsia during a previous pregnancy?	1
If so, was it severe?	2
Have you ever given birth to an infant that was premature (born at 36 weeks or earlier) or that weighed less than 5 pounds?	1
More than once?	5
Have you ever given birth to an infant that weighed 9½ pounds or more?	1
More than once?	2
Have you ever gone into labor with the baby not positioned head first?	1
Have you ever had twins (or triplets)?	1
Are you Rh-negative *and* have you had a positive antibody test?	7

Questions about your current and past medical health

Are you anemic? If so, is your hematocrit between 25 and 32?	1
Is it less than 25?	2
Do you have sickle cell trait?	2
Sickle cell disease?	7
Do you have mild hypertension?	2
Severe hypertension?	7
Do you have heart disease that limits your activity mildly?	2
Severely?	7
Were you a diabetic before this pregnancy?	7
Did you develop diabetes during pregnancy?	3
Have you ever been treated for thyroid disease?	1
During this pregnancy?	7
Have you ever had gonorrhea, syphilis, or genital herpes?	1
During this pregnancy?	7
Have you had any bladder and kidney infections prior to this pregnancy?	1
Have you had any this pregnancy?	3
If so, did you have a fever over 100 degrees?	5
Have you ever been hospitalized for psychiatric reasons?	1

E. RISK ASSESSMENT WORKSHEET (Continued)

Questions about habits and nutrition

Do you smoke?	1
Do you drink alcohol (including beer or wine) nearly every day?	2
Have you regularly used any illegal or illicit drugs?	2
At the time you became pregnant, were you more than 20 percent above your ideal weight?	1
Did you weigh more than 200 pounds?	5
Were you more than 10 percent below ideal weight?	2
Do you suspect that your nutrition has been inadequate this pregnancy?	3

Questions about this pregnancy

Is this your first pregnancy?	1
At the time of delivery, will you be 15 years of age or younger?	2
Will you be aged 35 or more?	2
Are you unmarried?	1
Did you first seek prenatal care later than 22 weeks, or will you have made fewer than five prenatal visits before delivery?	2
Total	_____

A total score of seven or greater puts your pregnancy in the high-risk category.

If you do fall in the high-risk group, you should discuss this with your health-care provider. Babies of high-risk pregnancies have more than four times the chance of developing serious medical problems or of dying than babies in low-risk pregnancies. It is important to recognize, however, that most high-risk mothers have good pregnancies and give birth to normal, healthy babies. Thus, identifying someone as being at relatively high risk does not mean there will in fact be problems with the pregnancy; it alerts the individual and her health-care provider that special care should be taken.

If you found yourself in the low-risk category, you should feel encouraged.

Looking ahead, some of the most significant information about risk of complications is not available before labor begins or until later on in labor. If you wish to continue to estimate your risk of complications, look over the page you have just completed when you go into labor, noting any changes that have occurred by that time. Then add to that score your responses to the following questions:

Additional Questions for Estimating Risk When Labor Begins

	Points
Are you less than 37 weeks pregnant, or is the baby estimated to weigh less than five pounds?	7
Are you more than 42 weeks pregnant?	7
Is the baby turned some other way than head down?	7
Do you have polyhydramnios (a large excess of amniotic fluid)?	7
Do you have mild preeclampsia?	3
Severe preeclampsia?	7
Do you have twins?	7
Did you gain less than 12 pounds this pregnancy?	5
Did you gain more than 48 pounds this pregnancy?	3
Total	_____

Once again, a total score of seven or above (including your score for the risk assessment at mid-pregnancy) puts your pregnancy in the high-risk category.

Careful assessment of risk factors is an important part of prenatal care given by doctors, midwives, and other medical personnel. The questions listed above can help you understand something about how such an assessment is done and about the relative risk of your own pregnancy.

If you ended up in the high-risk group, we hope you were not unduly alarmed; nearly half of all pregnant women are at high risk by this system, and most of them do quite well. If you have few or no risk factors, your labor will still need to be observed carefully, because a large percentage of complications of labor (nearly a third) occur in women thought to be at relatively low risk.

F. WORKSHEET FOR ESTIMATING YOUR DUE DATE

Event	Date	Week of pregnancy	Estimated due date by this method
Start of last menstrual period	_____	0	_____
Conception (if you know date)	_____	2	_____
Physician or midwife's estimate of pregnancy duration at first prenatal visit	_____		_____
First awareness of fetal movement	_____	17–19 (first baby)	_____
	_____	15–17 (second baby)	_____
Ultrasound (if done)	_____		_____

G. YOUR FOOD DIARY

The two-day food diary on the next two pages gives you a way to look carefully at your pregnancy diet and to pinpoint changes you need to make. Fill out the diary by writing down *everything* you eat for two days, from when you wake up in the morning until you go to sleep at night. Be sure to include all snacks and all drinks.

Suggestions for using the food diary:

1. Look at *each* item of food you have recorded, and write next to it the number of the food group to which it belongs. Some foods, such as cereal with fruit and milk, or a vegetable-and-rice casserole, will represent several food groups. Be sure to note this.

2. Count the times each food group is represented each day, and compare your totals with the recommendations on page 40.

3. Put a checkmark by items that have little or no food value or that are high in sugar, fat, and calories.

4. Star those foods that are "nutrient-dense."

5. Look over your diet and decide where you can make changes that will improve your nutrition. For instance, replace high-calorie or fat foods with those that are nutrient-dense, processed foods with whole grains, juices with sodas, etc.

6. Now write down your goals for changing your diet, and start right away to make changes. You can list your goals on the page following the entries for your food diary.

7. In one week, fill out another food diary to check on yourself. You should see much improvement.

DAY ONE

Date: _____

MORNING

Time   Foods

_____   _____

_____   _____

_____   _____

_____   _____

_____   _____

_____   _____

_____   _____

MID-DAY

Time   Foods

_____   _____

_____   _____

_____   _____

_____   _____

_____   _____

_____   _____

EVENING

Time   Foods

_____   _____

_____   _____

_____   _____

_____   _____

_____   _____

_____   _____

DAY TWO

Date: _____

MORNING:

Time   Foods

_____   _____

_____   _____

_____   _____

_____   _____

_____   _____

_____   _____

MID-DAY

Time   Foods

_____   _____

_____   _____

_____   _____

_____   _____

_____   _____

EVENING

Time   Foods

_____   _____

_____   _____

_____   _____

_____   _____

_____   _____

_____   _____

GOALS:

1. _____

_____

_____

_____

_____

_____

2. _____

_____

_____

_____

_____

_____

3. _____

_____

_____

_____

_____

_____

4. _____

_____

_____

_____

_____

_____

5. _____

_____

_____

_____

_____

_____

H. CHART YOUR OWN WEIGHT GAIN

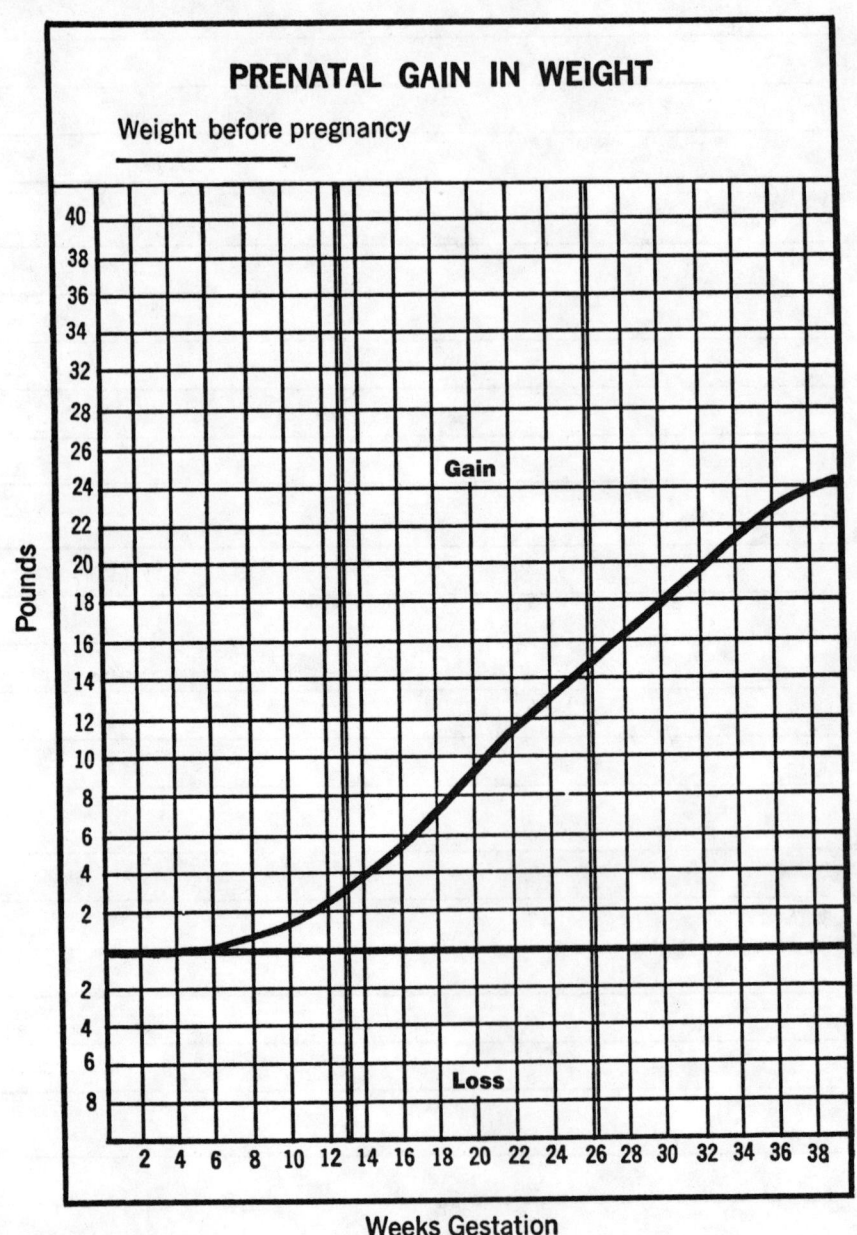

This chart shows the average weight gain in pregnancy. You can chart your own weight gain here and see how you compare.

I. YOUR FITNESS DIARY

Week	Stretching (daily)	Kegels (daily)	Abdominal strengthening exercises (3–5 times / week)	Aerobic exercise (3–5 times / week)	Relaxation (daily)

I. YOUR FITNESS DIARY (Continued)

	Week	Stretching (daily)	Kegels (daily)	Abdominal strengthening exercises (3—5 times / week)	Aerobic exercise (3—5 times / week)	Relaxation (daily)

J. YOUR PRESCRIPTIONS AND OVER-THE-COUNTER DRUGS

Prescriptions

List *all* prescription drugs you take regularly, all you take once in a while, and all that you have around the house or in your purse even though you no longer take them. Include drugs for birth control (even foams and jellies), pain pills, allergy medicines, antibiotics, skin preparations, and so on.

Drug name	What it's used for	How often taken	Taken this pregnancy? (approx. dates)

Over-the-Counter Drugs

Now list all the over-the-counter drugs you have around the house, including all vitamins, drugs such as aspirin or Tylenol, antacids, sunscreens, pills for menstrual cramps, medicated skin creams, old remedies, and so on.

Drug name	What it's used for	How often taken	Taken this pregnancy? (approx. dates)

K. YOUR SOCIAL DRUGS

Item	Yes	No	How much and how often
coffee	☐	☐	_____
tea	☐	☐	_____
soft drinks containing caffeine, such as Tab and Coke	☐	☐	_____
herb teas (specify)	☐	☐	_____
alcohol (specify)	☐	☐	_____
cigarettes	☐	☐	_____
other tobacco	☐	☐	_____
marijuana	☐	☐	_____
other recreational or street drugs	☐	☐	_____

L. A PROGRAM FOR QUITTING SMOKING

You know that smoking is one of the worst things you can do for yourself and your baby. But you also know that it can be very difficult to quit. There's no doubt about it, it's hard to break the habit. *But it can be done.* Most smokers who quit (95 percent) do so on their own. And now is the time, if there ever was one, for you to quit. Here is a method, called behavior modification or "self-directed change," that works for many people. (It can also be used to change other habitual behavior.) The steps outlined here are described in a book by John W. Farquhar, M.D., called *The American Way of Life Need Not Be Hazardous to Your Health* (New York: Norton, 1979). Carry out the six steps, in the order given, as many times as you need to.

Step 1. **Identify the problem.** Nicotine is harmful to my baby and myself, so I will quit smoking.

Step 2. **Build your confidence and commitment to quit.** You have identified the problem. Now become aware of when you smoke, and think about cutting down and quitting. Start by smoking one for every two or three cigarettes you would normally smoke. If you have trouble sticking with your commitment, recognize the negative speeches that go on inside your head.

Step 3. **Increase your awareness of why, when, and where you smoke.** Analyze why you smoke, what triggers your desire to smoke, and the reasons you give yourself for having a cigarette. Look at ways you can change your environment to help you be a nonsmoker: if you eat lunch with someone who always lights up after the meal, start eating with someone else, somewhere else. Better yet, convince your friend to join in your pact.

Step 4. **Build an Action Plan for Successful Quitting.** Write a contract that will cover a few weeks. It can look like the one on page 256 or you can develop your own. The contract should include people who will help you and ways you will reward yourself for not smoking. If you can't quit cold turkey, taper for a week or two, then try quitting. Tapering lets you practice suppressing the urge to smoke. Some people use relaxation to help suppress the urge.

Step 5. **Evaluate your program as time passes.** How effective is it? Are you achieving your goals? Any problem areas? Change the parts of the program that aren't working.

Step 6. **Maintain your program.** You have the best possible reason to maintain your nonsmoking: your future baby's health. Keep up the good work! If you backslide, start over with Step One.

SELF-CONTRACT TO QUIT SMOKING

Date _____

    To stop smoking, I will ask _____ to be my helper. I plan to quit smoking over a three-week period by cutting down the number of cigarettes I smoke by _____ a day until I reach zero level. I will use relaxation, exercise, and all the support I can get to help ease my desire to smoke.

    I will record the number of cigarettes I smoke per day, the number of times I call on my helper, and the number of times I divert myself by exercising or by other means.

    My helper agrees to talk to me every day to give me encouragement and support. At the end of three weeks my helper and I will review my contract.

    I will reward myself for not smoking by _____

_____

_____

_____

_____

Signed _____

Helper _____

M. WORK HISTORY

Both the expectant mother and the expectant father should fill this form out. Show it to your health-care provider.

Expectant Mother _____   Expectant Father _____

Date _____

Current Work List job title and date when you started the job; describe the work you do.

Mother: _____   Father: _____

_____   _____

_____   _____

_____   _____

_____   _____

History of Exposures

List *any* known or suspected exposures to any of the substances in table 4 (pages 76–77) and exposures to any other substances that concern you. Note any effects you feel may have been caused by them.

Mother: _____

_____

_____

_____

_____

Father: _____

_____

_____

_____

Family Exposures

Does anyone in your family work in a job that could involve bringing hazardous substances home? Has anyone in the past? Consider such substances as asbestos, lead, beryllium, and vinyl chloride. Also, list any possibly hazardous substances related to housework, home crafts, and hobbies.

Mother: _____

_____

_____

_____

_____

Father: _____

_____

_____

257

N. PRENATAL SUMMARY FOR TRAVELERS

Your name _____ Birth date ____ / ____ / ____

Prenatal care provided by _____ phone (____) _____

In case of emergency notify _____ phone (____) _____

Date of last menstrual period ____ / ____ / ____ Due date ____ / ____ / ____

Number of previous pregnancies _____

Major risk factors _____

_____

Summary of laboratory work

Blood type _____ Rh _____

Hematocrit   date ____ / ____ / ____   result _____

_____ / ____ / ____   _____

_____ / ____ / ____   _____

Ultrasound (if done)   date ____ / ____ / ____

result _____

Prenatal visits

Date	Blood pressure	Uterine size (cm)	Urine	Comments
____	____ / ____	____	____ / ____	_____
____	____ / ____	____	____ / ____	_____
____	____ / ____	____	____ / ____	_____
____	____ / ____	____	____ / ____	_____
____	____ / ____	____	____ / ____	_____
____	____ / ____	____	____ / ____	_____
____	____ / ____	____	____ / ____	_____

O. A CHECKLIST OF THINGS YOU MAY WISH TO GET DONE BEFORE DELIVERY

☐ register and attend childbirth class (5th month)

☐ preregister at the hospital (8th month)

☐ prepare the nursery for the baby

☐ decide on bottle- or breastfeeding

☐ decide who will be with you during labor

☐ decide about circumcision (if it's a boy)

☐ agree on visitation schedule for relatives during first weeks after birth

☐ decide on diapering method; contact a diaper service if needed

☐ see printer about birth announcements

☐ prepare birth-announcement address list

☐ arrange for religious ceremonies

☐ pack your suitcase

☐ discuss with your health-care provider when and how to contact him or her

☐ double-check plans for getting to the hospital and for childcare during labor (if needed)

☐ prepare for breastfeeding by toughening your nipples (8th and 9th months)—see page 98

P. A CHECKLIST OF SUPPLIES FOR YOUR BABY

Feeding supplies

- ☐ bottles (8 oz. and 4.4 oz. sizes)
- ☐ nipples
- ☐ bottle brush*

  (the number of bottles and nipples will depend on whether you're bottle- or breast-feeding, or combining)

Furniture

- ☐ crib
- ☐ mattress
- ☐ crib bumpers
- ☐ cradle or bassinet
- ☐ rocking chair*
- ☐ changing table*
- ☐ playpen (you'll probably want one later if not now)

Bedding

- ☐ fitted crib sheets
- ☐ blankets
- ☐ receiving blankets
- ☐ quilted crib-size mattress pad
- ☐ large and small crib pads for over and under the sheet

Bath and grooming supplies

- ☐ plastic tub
- ☐ baby soap, shampoo, and lotion
- ☐ soft hair brush
- ☐ nail scissors
- ☐ corn starch (use instead of baby powder)
- ☐ wash cloths
- ☐ towels
- ☐ cotton balls

Clothing

- ☐ undershirts
- ☐ nightgowns
- ☐ sleepers (one piece with feet)
- ☐ sweaters, jacket, bonnets, mittens, etc. (depending on climate)

Diapering supplies

- ☐ cloth diapers
- ☐ waterproof pants
- ☐ diaper pins
- ☐ disposable wipes (or your own means of cleaning baby's bottom)
- ☐ ointment for diaper rash
- ☐ disposable diapers (even if you use cloth diapers, you'll want some on hand)

  (the number of diapers will depend on whether you plan to use a diaper service or disposable diapers, or wash your own; if you'll be washing, get two dozen)

Visual stimulation

- ☐ mobiles, pictures, toys

Traveling supplies

- ☐ car seat (make sure it meets all state and federal safety standards)**
- ☐ carriage and/or stroller
- ☐ baby carrying pack
- ☐ diaper and equipment bag

*Not absolutely necessary—but nice.

**About car seats: Every state except Wyoming requires infants and young children to be transported in *approved* safety seats. For information and recommendations on car seats, contact your state's Highway Safety Program or the National Child Passenger Safety Program (215-642-4360). Many communities have rental programs for approved safety seats. Contact your local health department for information.

Q. A CHECKLIST OF THINGS TO TAKE TO THE HOSPITAL*

☐ Things that remind you of home, such as a tape player with your favorite music, and your own clothing.

☐ A watch with a second hand, for timing contractions.

☐ Books to read while in early labor.

☐ Two pairs of warm socks. Feet are often cold in labor, and warm socks will help you relax.

☐ Baby powder or corn starch, for massage. Empty a shaker-topped bottle (such as a spice bottle), clean it, and fill it with the powder.

☐ A small bottle of baby oil, for perineal massage.

☐ Pillows. Extra pillows are often helpful for positioning. If you use colored pillowcases, they won't get lost.

☐ A rolling pin or tennis ball to provide counter-pressure and to massage the back during back labor. Particularly useful are the plastic rolling pins that are hollow and can be filled with warm water.

☐ Lollipops.

☐ Notes for the coach, to remind him or her of the basics of labor and support (see pages 262–63).

☐ Toothbrush and toothpaste.

☐ Rubber bands and hairbrush. If your hair is long, braiding it will keep you cooler and prevent tangles.

☐ A camera with flash or indoor film (preset for people who aren't familiar with it).

☐ A focal point that is simple, pleasant, and portable, and masking tape to tape it to the wall.

☐ Food for dad or the friend who will be your coach: a thermos of coffee (or tea or soup), lots of sandwiches and homemade cookies (wrapped and frozen in advance), and fresh fruit. Some food for you, too, in case you have the baby at night and find yourself very hungry.

☐ Razor, toothbrush, and toothpaste for dad.

☐ A list, with phone numbers, of people to call with the news.

☐ A nightgown that opens in front, for nursing mothers. Nursing bra, underwear, too.

☐ Sanitary napkins.

☐ Special clothes to take the baby home in.

*Adapted from a list by Lisa Goldstein, Burnsville, N.C.

R. NOTES FOR THE COACH TO REFER TO DURING LABOR

Stage of labor	What happens	What you may notice in the mother	What to do
Latent phase	• Mild contractions • Cervix effaces & dilates to 3 cm • May last many hours	• Contractions become regular • Contractions go from 30 min. apart to every 6–8 min. • Mother is excited, confident, talkative • Slow, rhythmic breathing needed with some contractions	• Encourage restful activities • Have mother empty bladder every hr. • Time & record contractions • Help in breathing, use focal point, massage (if needed)
Early active phase	• Contractions intensify • Cervix dilates from 3 to 7 cm • Lasts up to several hrs.	• Contractions every 3–5 min. • Mother needs to concentrate, to breath with contractions	• Help mother breathe and concentrate during contractions • Have her use cleansing breath and relax between • Control pain with massage, back pressure, compresses, positioning • Have mother keep mouth moist, empty bladder every hour

Notes from childbirth classes

_____

_____

_____

_____

_____

_____

_____

R. NOTES FOR THE COACH TO REFER TO DURING LABOR (Continued)

Stage of labor	What happens	What you may notice in the mother	What to do
Transition	• Contractions *very* intense • Cervix dilates from 7 to 10 cm. • Lasts up to an hour or two	• Mother appears irritable, on edge • Shivering, nausea, & vomiting are common • Mother fatigued between contractions • Urge to push begins to develop	• Help mother make it through each contraction individually • Remember—this phase is short • Help her relax between contractions • Don't leave her alone • Help her with breathing techniques
Second stage (pushing)	• Contractions & mother's effort push baby down through vagina • Ends with birth	• Pushing requires great effort by mother, but comes as a relief • Learning to push effectively can take a while • Contractions are a little less frequent	• Assist mother to position herself comfortably • Help with pushing by encouraging her • Relax her between contractions • Use cool compresses • Get camera ready (if pictures are desired)
Birth of baby & afterwards	• Baby is born • Placenta comes out (usually within 20 min. of baby) • Episiotomy & lacerations are repaired	• Mother is excited & fatigued • Sense of relief & calm • Uncontrollable shaking (normal after birth)	• Help with breathing as needed • Hold baby • Assist mother with baby • Take pictures

Notes from childbirth classes

_____

_____

_____

_____

_____

S. DELIVERY AND BIRTH INFORMATION CHARTS

Here are two charts on which you can record the basic details of your childbirth. The delivery information chart includes the information most important for the mother's records. The birth information chart includes the information most important for the baby's records.

Delivery Information Chart

Hospital or birthing center _____

Date of delivery _____ Time _____

Doctor or midwife _____

Labor nurse _____

Medications taken _____

Length of labor _____

Labor complications _____

_____

Birth Information Chart

Date of birth _____ Time _____

Hospital or birthing center _____

Apgar scores _____ at 1 min. _____ at 5 min.

Birth weight _____ pounds _____ grams

Length _____ inches _____ centimeters

Head circumference _____

Blood type/Rh: _____

Pediatrician or family doctor _____

Neonatal complications _____

Index